SELF-HELP
HANDBOOK
OF SYMPTOMS
AND TREATMENTS

JOEL N. SHLIAN, M.D.
DEBORAH M. SHLIAN, M.D.

CONTEMPORARY
BOOKS, INC.
CHICAGO ▪ NEW YORK

Library of Congress Cataloging-in-Publication Data

Shlian, Joel N.
  Self-help handbook of symptoms and treatments.

  1. Self-care, Health.   2. Consumer education.
I. Shlian, Deborah M.   II. Title.   III. Title: Self-
help handbook of symptoms and
treatments.   [DNLM: 1. Medicine—popular works.
2. Self Care—popular works.   WB 120 S558s]
RA776.95.S54   1986   616   86-2597
ISBN 0-8092-5146-9 (pbk.)

Editorial director: Duane R. Carlson,
                    Vice-President, Communications,
                    Blue Cross and Blue Shield Association

Text illustrations: Sam Thiewes

Published by Contemporary Books, Inc.
180 North Michigan Avenue, Chicago, Illinois 60601
Manufactured in the United States of America
Library of Congress Catalog Card Number: 86-2597
International Standard Book Number: 0-8092-5146-9

Published simultaneously in Canada by Beaverbooks, Ltd.
195 Allstate Parkway, Valleywood Business Park
Markham, Ontario L3R 4T8 Canada

Note to Readers

This book is intended as a symptom-oriented consumer health guide. While every effort has been made to provide clear and accurate information, no book can be a substitute for an actual medical evaluation of particular signs or symptoms. Symptoms and treatments included here are discussed in only a general way and the reader must recognize that these discussions and recommendations may not apply in every case. This book is not intended in any manner as a substitute for careful medical diagnosis and treatment of symptoms and underlying illnesses.

Other books in **Your Healthy Best** series

Guide to More Healthful Living
Personal Fitness Diary

Authors' note: For ease of reading, we have used the masculine pronoun when referring to your physician or medical specialist. This is in no way intended to slight or offend female medical professionals but is meant only to allow economy of words.

Contents

SELF-HELP HANDBOOK
OF SYMPTOMS
AND TREATMENTS

Introduction

You want to be healthy and fit. You aren't alone.

More people than ever not only want good health, they go to considerable effort to achieve it. Men and women all around you are exercising, keeping trim, and coming to terms with the stresses in their lives. People are smoking less, eating better, and even fastening their seat belts.

You now go through life immunized from infectious diseases like measles, diphtheria, and whooping cough. You can benefit from spectacular new medical advances that make it possible to cure some forms of cancer, transplant vital organs, and replace damaged bones and joints.

A child born today in the United States can expect to live well over 70 years. That's a longer life expectancy than was possible in any previous generation, and during those 70 or more years, Americans can enjoy the highest standard of health ever known.

This book complements your quest for a healthy life. It gives you information on what to do when your health is not at its best. It is a fundamental guide to many common symptoms that may indicate problems, and it indicates the steps to take to protect your health when problems arise.

1

Part I opens with important background information to help you become a wise health care consumer. It gives you tips on how to select a doctor and when to seek his advice. It gives you helpful hints for dealing with modern-day hazards like overeating, alcohol and drug abuse, and stress. It also contains advice for travelers and senior citizens.

Parts II and III make this book particularly useful by focusing on symptoms you may experience. To use other manuals effectively, you have to know or at least suspect a particular disease before you can understand your symptoms or consider taking any action. For example, if your hip hurts, you might look under *osteoarthritis*— among other hip diseases—to determine if it may be affecting you. This book takes an easier approach. If your hip hurts, you look up the symptoms and read about the possible causes and complications that should concern you. We think that is simpler than having to look up osteoarthritis first and then find out whether it is the cause of your problem.

Part II contains a broad discussion of symptoms that may affect the entire body. Part III covers particular symptoms that indicate conditions in specific parts of the body.

Together, these two parts will give you both the broad and narrow perspectives on matters affecting your health. If your hip hurts, for example, you can first get an overview of the problem from Part II in the section "Generalized Bone and Joint Swelling and Pain." From there you can turn to Part III and consult the section "Symptoms and Diseases Affecting the Bones, Joints, and Muscles." Then, within this section, you can focus specifically on hip ailments in the subsection "Hip Pain and Symptoms."

Part IV, "Symptoms and Diseases of Children," focuses on areas of particular concern to parents—a quick reference to the most common symptoms in young children.

Finally, Part V highlights "Common Medical Emergencies," the types of accidents and sudden illnesses that require prompt and immediate action. This section tells you how to recognize and respond to such emergency situations.

Each section on a particular set of symptoms is divided into four parts. The first part, labeled "Description," is exactly that—a general description of the symptoms that you might encounter and what they generally indicate. The part entitled "When To Be Concerned" tells you when your symptoms mean you need to see your doctor and how

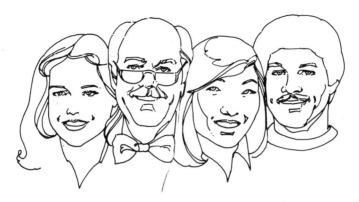

urgently you need his care. A recommendation simply to seek medical attention generally means you should make an appointment and see the doctor within a few days. When *prompt* attention is recommended, you need care within a day, and *immediate* attention means just that—get medical help right now. You should seek immediate care whenever you have any suspicion that you are in an emergency situation.

The third part of each section is entitled "Treatment." Here you'll read about home remedies you can use when you are suffering from a condition that is not serious enough to require professional care or when there are home measures you can take *before* seeking professional care. Sometimes, when such home treatment is successful, you will not need to see your doctor; other times, you will be urged to follow up such treatment with a visit to your physician whether or not the treatment appears to have been successful. This "Treatment" discussion also tells you how the doctor will diagnose and treat a condition that requires his care, and it prepares you for the questions the doctor may ask in evaluating your symptoms.

Finally, each section concludes with a list entitled "Call Your Doctor When." This list is intended to serve as a reference to help you quickly identify those symptoms that require medical care. So that you can easily identify the symptoms that represent emergencies or situations urgently requiring medical attention, the phrase *call immediately* follows certain symptoms, in italics and in parentheses. If you are unable to reach your doctor, do not delay in seeking care at your local hospital emergency room.

Often, a symptom you notice may be accompanied by other symptoms, or other areas of the body may be affected in some way by the cause of your symptom. To avoid repeating information, we have included cross-references, where appropriate, to other sections of the book that contain information pertinent to your symptoms. To locate these other sections, use the index at the back of the book.

This book is organized to provide easy reference to medical information. You start with a symptom, and the book discusses its treatment with a minimum of reading. This can be a major factor in helping you stay healthy and fit.

Good luck and good health!

PART I

KEYS TO GOOD
HEALTH

Chapter 1

Your Relationship with Your Doctor

HOW TO FIND THE RIGHT DOCTOR

Today, finding a doctor is hardly an easy task. Long gone are the days when you simply called your neighborhood general practitioner for all your family's routine care. Modern medicine is practiced in a bewildering array of specialties. Doctors are more likely to practice in groups that may contain more than a hundred physicians in a dozen or more specialties.

Today, you are looking for a doctor to be your primary care physician—someone to solve most of your medical problems and to direct you to the proper specialist when necessary. Your primary doctor may be a pediatrician, a family practitioner, or an internist. He will take care of 90 percent of your routine medical problems.

How do you find the right doctor? There are three qualities that will determine how much trust you place in him: competence, concern, and compatibility. By *competence*, we mean that your doctor must be a skilled professional. By *concern*, we mean not only should he care for you, he also should care *about* you. By *compatibility*, we mean the doctor should be a person you like, someone with whom you can comfortably discuss intimate details of your life. As a practical matter, you may want to add *convenience,* meaning your doctor will be nearby and accessible so you can get to him readily when you need him.

Start looking for this doctor before you need him, when you are feeling well and can search objectively. Search by asking people very seriously which doctors are competent, compatible, and convenient. You can ask friends, relatives, neighbors, people you meet at parties, people you work with. You can ask the company doctor at your place of employment. You can ask doctors in other specialties. If you are new in town and don't know anyone, ask the doctor who cared for you in the town you left.

Another source is the referral service of the local medical society. You can get the names of two or three doctors who are taking on new patients. You can also call hospitals and get the names of internists and family practitioners on staff.

Sourcebooks are also available to help you. The *AMA Directory of Physicians* lists doctors by name, city, state, and medical specialties. The *Directory of Medical Specialists* lists the teaching affiliations of all doctors who have passed recognized specialty boards. Both of these books are updated regularly and are available in public libraries.

Where a doctor was trained and served his residency can give you additional insight into his competence: the best training is often in university hospitals. Doctors take pride in their years of academic training, and most will gladly discuss them with you.

Several factors can affect your final choice. One is recommendations. Those from laypeople are more subjective; recommendations from medical people are more authoritative but less freely given. However, you can assume that the more positive recommendations you get for a particular doctor, the more dependable those recommendations will be. Well-established reputations are often well-deserved.

Some find that a personal visit is the key to making a decision. You can evaluate the doctor and his support staff in a situation unclouded by the tension of a serious illness.

Be up front about your search. Tell the doctor you are looking for a physician and ask to see him for a blood pressure check or for an immunization update. You can evaluate the doctor's "bedside manner" as well as observe what he does himself and what he delegates to an assistant. You can judge the friendliness of the office staff, and you can make that very important compatibility determination. You will have the opportunity to talk to the doctor about availability, hospital privileges, charging practices, and whether he accepts assignment for Medicare or participates in the particular health insurance plan in which you are enrolled. It will cost you the price of a regular office visit, which probably will be a sound investment in your future and your medical care.

Remember, by becoming a partner in your medical care, you reap the benefits of better health and increased satisfaction.

WHEN TO SEEK A DOCTOR'S ADVICE

Now that you have chosen your primary care physician, when do you seek this doctor's medical advice?

Many people think they need to see the doctor for an annual physical examination, but you probably won't need a complete exam each year if you are between 20 and 40 and in good health. Annual checkups are expensive and time-consuming. They may even give you a false sense of security, leading you to think you are healthy and possibly causing you to ignore a sudden symptom that signals the need for immediate care.

Instead, your doctor may suggest periodic health screening. Depending on your age, work, family history, environment, and other risk factors, your doctor will decide how often certain tests are necessary. Some guidelines that many doctors follow include a yearly check for glaucoma for everyone over age 40. Women should have periodic Pap smears, with specific conditions determining the interval between them.

Beyond periodic screening, you may have symptoms that suggest a visit to the doctor. Ultimately, you will be the judge of when to seek medical advice, and this book can give you some general guidelines to help you make an intelligent decision.

Some symptoms are a clear cause for alarm and require *immediate* medical help. Go to the nearest emergency facility as soon as possible. You shouldn't even lose time trying to contact your doctor, whose office may not be equipped to treat some emergencies.

Emergency symptoms include loss of consciousness, hemorrhage, crushing chest pain, severe shortness of breath, and acute allergic reactions, among others.

This book is about symptoms and their meanings. It gives you basic, general guidelines by which you can recognize symptoms and understand enough about them to decide whether or not they suggest disorders serious enough to warrant your doctor's care. This book will *not* qualify you to analyze symptoms and make medical diagnoses. That will always be the job of your doctor.

In general, you should also avoid referring yourself to medical specialists. Your primary care physician can treat perhaps 90 percent of your ailments, and he can best direct you to the specialists qualified to treat the remaining 10 percent. He knows their work, he knows your needs, and he can best coordinate your health care with them.

Chapter 2

Positive Health Care

You want to be healthy and fit. Your doctor is responsible for your health and fitness, but so are you. When you adopt a healthy lifestyle and put yourself in the care of a physician, you and your doctor become partners in your good health. To fulfill your end of the partnership, you must gear your lifestyle to positive health care. This involves staying informed so that you can avoid well-known risks and adopt beneficial habits.

AVOIDING THE RISKS

SMOKING

Smoking is one of the most serious health hazards we face, and it is an avoidable one: *simply don't smoke*. Information on the many ways that smoking can put you at risk of serious health problems has been disseminated widely in recent years. If you're still not convinced, however, that smoking is dangerous, read the following list.

Nonsmokers:
- have only a twentieth of a smoker's chances of being one of the 100,000 people who die of lung cancer each year. They also are less

11

likely to develop cancer of the bladder, larynx, pancreas, and mouth.

• are two to three times less likely to die of heart disease. Their arteries are unconstricted by nicotine, and their blood pressure is less likely to rise.

• are not causing anyone to inhale secondhand smoke, which itself is hazardous, according to many experts.

• face less risk of spontaneous abortion and miscarriage. Nonsmoking women probably will give birth to larger, healthier children who will have lower risk of lung infection during the first year of life.

Some smokers think they are safe if they smoke only low-tar, low-nicotine brands. Not true! Even those brands put you at substantial risk of getting lung disease. In fact, you're likely to smoke more of these brands and thus get just as much tar and nicotine as you would from stronger cigarettes.

CONSIDERING QUITTING?

You can do it! Most authorities agree that quitting "cold turkey" works far better than trying to taper off gradually. This means breaking an addiction and enduring withdrawal symptoms of irritability, nervousness, diarrhea, nausea, and headache. It's not easy, but many people do it successfully, often even after repeated failures.

If you need help, contact the American Cancer Society (90 Park Avenue, New York, NY 10016).

ALCOHOL

Like smoking, alcohol can cause major health problems. However, the important factor is *how much* you drink. Only 1 in 20 people is a "problem drinker" or alcoholic, and those who drink moderately or not at all are at much less risk of alcohol-related health problems.

Moderate drinkers and abstainers:
• do not share the heavy drinker's serious risk of chronic liver inflammation, which leads to cirrhosis in at least 15 percent of all cases.

- are less likely to suffer from alcohol-related problems such as ulcers; pancreatic, kidney, and heart disease; neurological disorders; mental deterioration; paralysis of eye movements; and loss of touch and balance.
- avoid the metabolic problems that are caused by excess alcohol— lower levels of sugar and higher levels of fat in the blood, as well as elevated levels of acid in the body.
- are not likely to suffer interactions of alcohol with other medications, which kill several thousand people a year, and do not need to worry about diagnostic test results being distorted by alcohol.

Get Help for a Drinking Problem

Whether the problem is yours or a loved one's, there's only one way to tackle it: first, you must recognize the problem, then you must seek help. Fortunately, you have many resources to draw on. Programs and support groups are available in the community and in some companies. Alcoholics Anonymous is the largest and best known of these groups, with more than 10,000 groups meeting regularly throughout the country. Check your local Yellow Pages or ask your doctor for a referral to a local group.

STRESS

What exactly is stress? The word originally was used to describe your body's response to danger. You know it as a pounding heart and a surge of adrenaline in the face of a physical threat. Now the word has grown to mean much more. Sources of stress are emotional as well as physical. And the long-term effects are now being taken into account.

Stress-related illnesses have become significant problems in our society. Research has shown that heart disease, ulcers, high blood pressure, and migraine headaches are among the many disorders linked to stress. Stress also leads to increased use of drugs, alcohol, coffee, and tobacco.

So what can you do about stress? First understand that it is part of life. Then learn techniques of stress management.

Try to recognize when you are in stressful situations and observe how you react. You may bite your nails, tap your foot, crack your knuckles, or feel a stiffness in your neck or back. You might find yourself using the bathroom more often or blinking your eyes a lot. You might notice a muscle twitch.

The simplest method of stress management is simply to avoid stressful situations whenever you can. And when you can't avoid them, be creative in minimizing their effect on you:

- Take an exercise break. You may be able to relieve your tension with a few minutes of stretching or a quick dash up several flights of stairs. On your lunch hour, try more structured exercises like long walks or dance classes.
- Breathe. Inhale deeply and exhale slowly with your eyes closed. Forget house chores and office deadlines for just a moment and relax.

Make a habit of using techniques like these, and when you are ill, tell the doctor about the stresses you have been under. He will make a much better diagnosis when he allows for stress factors.

POSITIVE MEASURES TO PROTECT YOUR HEALTH

GOOD NUTRITION

In the simplest terms, good nutrition is essential to good health. But you must not confuse good nutrition with simply taking vitamins or eating sparingly to stay thin. You could be cheating yourself out of the balanced diet you need.

The fact is, you don't get good nutrition just from vitamin supplements. You get it from the four major food groups: meats, fruits and vegetables, bread, and milk. You balance your diet by eating healthful amounts from all of these groups—not too much and not too little of any. Each group supplies necessary nutrients:

- The meat group includes not only beef, pork, poultry, and fish but also things like eggs, beans, and peanuts. They are sources of protein, iron, zinc, and vitamins of the B complex.
- The fruit and vegetable group provides 90 percent of the vitamin C and at least 60 percent of the vitamin A you need. Fruits and vegetables also supply minerals, folic acid, and carbohydrates.

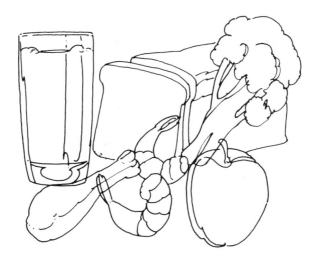

- The bread group, which includes cereals, is a source of carbohydrates, protein, thiamine, riboflavin, niacin, and iron.
- The milk group—including ice cream, yogurt, and cheese—is your main supplier of calcium, plus vitamin A, vitamin D, and many of the B vitamins.

The table on page 16 gives examples of foods in each group.

If you are like most Americans, you probably should cut down on caffeine and increase your intake of fiber. With less caffeine, you may lower your risk of heart disease and high blood pressure; if you are a woman, you will be at less risk of cystic breast cancer, and if you are pregnant, you will give your child a better chance against birth defects.

With a high-fiber diet (bran is recommended), you will increase bowel regularity and perhaps help prevent hemorrhoids, cancer of the bowel, and hardening of the arteries.

Another concern of today, based on the connection between a high intake of fats and cardiovascular disease, is the reduction of fats in our diets. A list of fat-containing foods is on page 17.

A Balanced Diet

Your well-balanced diet should consist of the four basic food groups. Select a wide variety of foods from within these categories. If you require a special diet because of a particular illness or during pregnancy, your doctor will advise you.

Group	Provides
I. Fruits & Vegetables broccoli lettuce cabbage carrots beets grapes prunes citrus fruits peaches	carbohydrates protein vitamin A, B complex, C folic acid minerals (calcium, iron, potassium, sodium)
II. Bread, Cereal, Grains wheat rye rice	carbohydrates protein vitamin B complex thiamine, niacin, iron
III. Milk and Dairy **Products** cheese milk yogurt buttermilk	protein fat, carbohydrates calcium riboflavin, vitamin A
IV. Meats beef veal pork fish eggs legumes (peas, beans)	protein fat iron, trace elements vitamin B complex

Types of Fats

Polyunsaturated (lowers cholesterol levels)
sunflower oil
safflower oil
corn oil
cottonseed oil
fish
soybean oil

Monounsaturated (no effect on cholesterol levels)
poultry
vegetable shortening
peanut butter and peanut oil
olives and olive oil
avocados

Saturated (raises cholesterol levels)
chocolate
cheese
butter
coconut oil
meat
egg yolk
palm oil
milk

Try to:
1. decrease the amounts of butterfats, eggs, and other high-cholesterol foods.
2. replace high-fat dairy products with low-fat dairy products.
3. reduce the amounts of animal fats in your diet.
4. replace, wherever possible, foods containing saturated fats with others containing polyunsaturated fats.

PHYSICAL FITNESS

Think of physical fitness as an overall pattern of living. It requires good nutrition, cleanliness, proper medical and dental care. And it means making exercise a regular part of your life—a much larger commitment than a few stretches and sit-ups each morning.

Exercise is good for you, though experts disagree widely on how good. Some say it can be the answer to a broad range of your health problems. Others, equally authoritative, say its advantages are minimal. Still others cite its psychological benefits: exercise causes the brain to release endorphins, hormones that bring about feelings of well-being.

The most effective exercises are aerobic: simple, strenuous activities that increase your heart and respiratory rates. These include bicycling, jumping rope, swimming, and distance running, and they all must be sustained for long periods of time to be worthwhile.

As a rule of thumb, if you are in good health, your *maximal* exercise pulse rate should be about 220 minus your age. Your *actual* exercise pulse rate, which you sustain most of the time you are working out, should be about three-quarters as fast. Generally, you should exercise at least three times a week and maintain your proper exercise heart rate for about 20 minutes each time.

See your doctor before you begin any strenuous exercise program. He may give you a stress EKG or other tests to determine just how much exercise you are able to tolerate. If you are overweight, he will put you on a balanced diet and will set a goal weight for you to reach through both diet and exercise.

Don't expect to lose a lot of weight through exercise alone. The pounds you shed from fat tissue tend to be supplanted by new pounds of muscle tissue. Exercise will help you control your appetite, however, and so will bring about weight loss indirectly.

IMMUNIZATIONS

When you are immunized—which you may think of as "getting your shots"—you receive probably the most worthwhile and cost-effective benefit of preventive health care.

Today, most children are properly immunized in the course of seeing their doctors regularly. But there still are many adults who did

Childhood Schedule of Immunizations, Skin Tests, and Boosters (Recommended by the American Academy of Pediatrics)

2 months	DPT*
	POLIO (TOPV)**
4 months	DPT
	POLIO (TOPV)
6 months	DPT
	POLIO (TOPV) (third shot optional—given only in high-risk areas)
12 months	Tuberculin Skin Test
15 months	Measles
	Mumps
	Rubella (German measles)
18 months	DPT
	POLIO (TOPV)
4-6 years	DPT
	POLIO (TOPV)
14-16 years	Diphtheria/Tetanus Toxoid (repeat every 10 years for life)

*Diphtheria, Pertussis (Whooping Cough), Tetanus
**Trivalent Oral Polio Vaccine

not receive childhood immunizations, and if you are one of them, you should consider getting your shots now—all except the pertussis (whooping cough) vaccine, which is not given after age six.

If you did receive immunizations as a child, you still need tetanus and diphtheria boosters every 10 years and additional tetanus shots whenever you suffer a wound that may become contaminated. Smallpox vaccinations are no longer needed. If you are a woman and planning to become pregnant, get a blood test to check whether you have antibodies against rubella (German measles). If these antibodies are not present, it means you have not had the disease and could catch it, and you should receive a rubella vaccination several months before becoming pregnant.

Many vaccines have been developed for adults, particularly those who are at high risk of complications from various diseases. Doctors may prescribe flu or pneumonia vaccines for patients who are elderly or suffer debilitating conditions like heart disease, diabetes, or chronic lung disease. Parents should be immunized against polio before their children, since the parents may be susceptible to the live virus in their children's vaccine.

The schedule of children's immunizations that precedes is recommended by the American Academy of Pediatrics. A single measles vaccination is now recommended at age 15 months. Children who were vaccinated before 12 months of age or who received inactivated vaccine should be revaccinated.

If you were born before 1957, you very likely have a natural immunity to measles. But if you were born after that date and received the inactivated vaccine used before 1968, you probably should ask your doctor about getting the current vaccine.

Consult a doctor for advice on all immunizations for both adults and children.

Chapter 3

Special Health Concerns

HEALTH CONCERNS
OF SENIOR CITIZENS

Because of the many advances in diagnosis and treatment of serious illness, you now stand a good chance of living well into your eighties, which means you could be spending many years as a senior citizen, dealing with the changes of later life. With a measure of understanding, you can make these truly the "golden years."

If someone in your household is a senior citizen, you probably have been made to realize that special problems come just with living longer. With aging, there is often decreased function of the heart, lungs, eyes, kidneys, and the musculoskeletal system—all of which make the elderly vulnerable to accidents, particularly falls. Poor vision most often causes accidents, and certain types of fractures often result.

You will go a long way toward preventing accidents simply by making your home safe. Keep the rooms well lit. Install handrails along the stairs and in the bathrooms.

You can look forward to being active in your old age. Many

community groups offer exercise programs and activities for the elderly. You will need to make a special effort to eat well: you must not fall into the habit of becoming careless about nutrition in old age. In particular, you will need adequate amounts of calcium to sustain bones and muscles.

In old age, depression can become a serious problem that you must be prepared to cope with. Don't resign yourself to it as something inevitable with advancing years. Keep a positive attitude and learn to enjoy every day. There is no reason why your senior years can't be the most worthwhile of all!

TIPS FOR HEALTHY TRAVEL

Many Americans can expect to travel, often to romantic and exotic places. And when you visit foreign lands, you want to guard against being visited in turn by foreign bacteria and parasites.

You will find that the old proverb—an ounce of prevention is worth a pound of cure—applies most aptly. Be sure the food you eat is well cooked: almost all bacteria and parasites are destroyed by cooking. Drink only carbonated bottled beverages and don't use ice.

Then, if, in spite of these precautions, you still develop diarrhea, turn to a clear-liquid diet of soups and juices. After 24 hours, add crackers and toast. If the symptoms persist or are especially severe, take bismuth subsalicylate (e.g., Pepto-Bismol) or paregoric.

Chances are you have only "traveler's diarrhea," and it will clear up after two days. But if the symptoms worsen, and you have high fever, chills, or bloody stools, seek *immediate* medical attention.

You often need immunizations before setting out, and each country sets its own requirements for the shots you must have. High-risk areas are Africa, India, southwestern Asia, and South America. In all of these, malaria remains a particular hazard.

Whenever you plan to travel in underdeveloped countries, you should be properly immunized against polio and should consider getting shots for typhoid, cholera, and hepatitis. Ask your travel agent which specific immunizations you will need in the countries you plan to visit or get the booklet *Health Information for Recreational Travel* from the U.S. Government Printing Office.

Wherever you go, take along antihistamines for colds and motion sickness and paregoric for diarrhea. Also take an adequate supply of your regular medications and a letter from your doctor summarizing your significant medical problems and allergies.

Finally, allow at least two or three days for your body to adjust to "jet lag," the drowsiness and irritability caused by disruption of your normal sleep schedule.

Have a wonderful, safe trip.

MEDICATIONS

If you look in your medicine cabinet, you'll probably find that you've accumulated dozens of over-the-counter preparations and the leftovers of several partly used prescriptions. This could be a dangerous assortment.

While the sunburn creams and lip balms are harmless enough, there is potential hazard in such nonprescription items as the anti-inflammatory drugs (such as aspirin, acetaminophen, ibuprofen), steroids for topical application (preparations containing cortisone or its derivatives), antibiotic creams, and strong cough suppressants. When you use these substances to treat yourself, you may be applying them to surface symptoms and masking the underlying diseases. Using a steroid cream on skin cancer, for instance, may relieve some symptoms but delay proper medical diagnosis and treatment.

Also, as you use more potent nonprescription drugs, you increase the risk of interactions between them and also of serious allergies.

When you use a drug in a course of home treatment, first read the package insert carefully, then watch closely for results. If your condition fails to improve, or if it worsens, see your doctor. Bring all the drugs you are using, nonprescription as well as those prescribed by other doctors.

Prescription drugs can be confusing. More and more of them have become available in recent years. When one is taken off the market, it is replaced by several others. One drug can have several different product names, and many are available in generic form.

Your doctor will prescribe drugs that he is familiar with so he can tell you what side effects to expect. He needs to know all the drugs you are taking, prescription and over-the-counter, so he will not prescribe one that will interact with another. Unless he tells you otherwise, take prescriptions for the prescribed length of time, even if your symptoms go away before that time is up. If you notice any side effects, call your doctor *immediately*. He will tell you whether or not to stop taking the medication and will change your prescription if necessary. Never, under any circumstances, take anyone else's medications.

As a general rule, you should not keep any prescription drugs that you aren't taking on a regular basis. Keep only those prescribed during the past year, but keep adequate supplies of the drugs you do take regularly. Finally, keep all medications in one place, labeled carefully, and out of the reach of children.

PART II

SYMPTOMS AFFECTING THE ENTIRE BODY

Chapter 4

General Symptoms

WEAKNESS, FATIGUE, AND EXHAUSTION

DESCRIPTION

Most of you probably feel tired when you say you are fatigued or exhausted, but what do you mean when you say you feel weak? It's important to understand the differences, since each symptom may have a completely separate cause. Fatigue and exhaustion are often the result of emotional upset, unusual stress, or just plain boredom. Since the cause is generally psychological, it often goes away with rest and a change of mood.

Prolonged feelings of fatigue may be an early sign of depression (*see* Depression). Many other symptoms often accompany this kind of fatigue, including trouble sleeping (insomnia) (*see* Sleep Disorders), headaches (*see* Headaches), sexual dysfunction, and irritability. On the other hand, chronic fatigue could be an early sign of heart or lung disease. Disorders such as heart failure and emphysema cause fatigue because they prevent adequate amounts of oxygen from reaching the blood and body tissues.

While fatigue and exhaustion have to do with feeling tired, true weakness means an actual loss of muscle strength (*see* Localized Weakness). Using special tests, your doctor can determine the location and severity of the weakness. Then he will be able to identify the cause and begin treatment.

We usually associate fatigue, exhaustion, and weakness with each other because they often occur together. Many times these are symptoms associated with such common illnesses as colds and flu (*see* Colds and Cough). On the other hand, they may accompany more serious diseases such as mononucleosis (*see* Sore Throat), hepatitis (*see* Nausea and Vomiting), various disorders of your endocrine glands such as diabetes (*see* Frequent Urination) or thyroid disease, certain nutritional deficiencies, and some diseases of the nervous system. Sometimes, fatigue or weakness may be associated with actual dizziness or fainting (*see* Dizziness, Vertigo, or Loss of Consciousness).

When you feel "tired all the time," it is important first to try to distinguish between chronic fatigue and actual muscle weakness. Fatigue is much more common. Once you determine that fatigue is your problem, carefully analyze your lifestyle. Are you eating properly and getting enough rest and exercise? Have you maintained your weight?

If your answer to these questions is yes, you must then analyze your psychological lifestyle. Is your family life happy? Are you satisfied with your job? Do you have regular activities that you enjoy? Are you generally relaxed? Remember that one of the most common causes of fatigue is stress.

WHEN TO BE CONCERNED

Whenever you experience prolonged fatigue that is unrelieved by normal diet and rest, you should seek medical advice. When your fatigue is accompanied by other symptoms, such as chest discomfort or shortness of breath, you should see your doctor *immediately*. The same is true if you develop weakness in your muscles.

TREATMENT

Treatment of your fatigue or muscle weakness is aimed at treating the underlying cause. If you are feeling tired and know it's because you're just not eating or sleeping properly, try to correct the situation. Follow a regular exercise program. If the fatigue persists with or without other symptoms, your doctor will need to evaluate the problem.

CALL YOUR DOCTOR WHEN:

- your fatigue is not relieved by normal diet and sleep.
- your fatigue is chronic and persists over several weeks.
- your fatigue is associated with loss or gain of more than a few pounds of weight.
- your fatigue is associated with other symptoms such as heart palpitations, shortness of breath, dizziness, fainting, severe headache, or fever.
- your fatigue is accompanied by severe depression.
- you experience true muscle weakness.

DIZZINESS, VERTIGO, OR LOSS OF CONSCIOUSNESS

DESCRIPTION

You probably have experienced the symptom of dizziness (*see* Dizziness). It can best be described as a sensation of unsteadiness or light-headedness. In some cases, it may be associated with a feeling of faintness. However, with dizziness, you do not actually faint or lose consciousness (*see* Loss of Consciousness). You may feel dizzy after having one drink too many or immediately after getting off an amusement park ride. Emotional upset and stress may sometimes produce this symptom.

Vertigo is often confused with simple dizziness, but it is generally a more serious medical symptom. Vertigo can best be described as an actual sense of movement. With vertigo, you perceive that either you or your surroundings are actually moving or spinning. When you try to walk, you may veer to one side.

Vertigo is usually the result of a disturbance in either the inner portion of your ear or certain areas of the brain responsible for maintaining your balance. Any acute or chronic disorder that affects the nerves leading to these areas can also cause vertigo. One of the most common causes is a mild viral illness associated with head and ear stuffiness. Sometimes the symptom of vertigo doesn't even appear until after the infection has cleared up. Typically, the symptom is worse when you turn your head or change positions (positional vertigo). More serious causes include head injury, drug overdose, and brain tumors.

A sudden loss of consciousness is called fainting. Fainting is usually a result of a sudden decrease in the blood supply to the brain. Many mechanisms can affect the blood flow to your brain, and some of these are part of your body's natural reaction to anxiety, particularly stress. The very act of fainting and falling down often increases the blood supply to your brain. Fatigue, hunger, and emotional stress are common causes of fainting.

WHEN TO BE CONCERNED

Although dizziness is generally nothing to worry about, it may be a clue to something more serious, such as hypoglycemia (low blood sugar), anemia, high or low blood pressure, drug overdose, or heart disease. Anytime you experience dizziness that does not go away within a fairly short time, consult your physician.

An occasional episode of vertigo that is short-lived should not be a cause for alarm. However, recurrent, frequent, severe attacks of vertigo require medical attention. Likewise, vertigo associated with head injury or accompanied by fainting requires immediate medical attention.

Most often, fainting is harmless except for the risk of head injury. Recovery from an uncomplicated episode of fainting should occur within minutes. Loss of consciousness may also accompany heart disease, severe anemia, diabetes, hypoglycemia, drug overdoses, and epilepsy. Any time someone loses consciousness and can't be aroused (coma), consider this a medical emergency and call for an ambulance.

TREATMENT

The treatment of dizziness, vertigo, or loss of consciousness depends on the cause of the symptom. If you have become dizzy because of an emotional upset or stress, often a brief period of rest and an attempt to eliminate the underlying cause will solve your problem. Vertigo that is a result of a mild viral illness will generally go away within a few days without treatment. If you become faint, lie down right away or sit with your head between your knees.

For recurrent dizziness, vertigo, or fainting episodes, your doctor will need to do a complete evaluation in order to prescribe appropriate therapy. He will need to determine the underlying cause and to be certain that there has been no head trauma or other injury if you have lost consciousness.

CALL YOUR DOCTOR WHEN:

- you experience dizziness that doesn't go away within a short time.
- you experience recurrent episodes of dizziness or vertigo.
- you experience dizziness, vertigo, or fainting associated with a head injury or convulsion (call immediately).
- you experience recurrent fainting episodes (call immediately).
- you are unable to arouse someone who is unconscious (call for an ambulance immediately).

FEVER WITH OR WITHOUT CHILLS

DESCRIPTION

Fever is probably the single most important symptom of illness. It is also one of the main ways in which your body defends itself against disease. Normally, oral body temperature ranges between 96.8 and 99.3 degrees Fahrenheit (normal rectal temperature is one degree higher). Like a built-in thermostat, a center in the brain keeps your temperature within this normal range in spite of conditions outside your body, such as hot weather or heavy clothing.

When you become sick, especially with a serious infection, the invading germs cause your body to produce substances that circulate to the brain center and reset this thermostat. As your body works to keep this higher temperature in order to help fight the infection, you feel feverish. Your fever may begin either with a sensation of flushing and warmth or with chills. Soon your pulse rate will increase, and you may experience aches and pains in your muscles.

Although infections are the most common cause of fever, anything that interferes with the thermostat in your brain can produce an elevated temperature, including stroke, cancer, heart attack, and an overactive thyroid gland (hyperthyroidism).

WHEN TO BE CONCERNED

An increased temperature is a clue that you may be ill. However, the number itself does not necessarily tell you how sick you are. In general, children tend to have higher fevers than adults, while elderly people may not have very high fevers even when they are quite ill. So how do you know when to be concerned? A low-grade fever (under 102 degrees Fahrenheit orally) associated with symptoms of cold or flu is generally no cause for alarm. However, if your fever increases beyond a low grade, or if there are other symptoms associated with your fever such as wet cough (*see* Cough and/or Shortness of Breath), severe shaking chills, unusually severe headache, or neck stiffness, consult your doctor. A prolonged low-grade fever, even without other symptoms, or a fever that comes and goes over a period of several weeks should also receive medical attention. Extremely high fevers, particularly in infants or young children, will occasionally cause convulsions (*see* Convulsions). This should be considered a medical emergency requiring immediate medical care.

TREATMENT

Because fever is simply a symptom and not a disease itself, treatment depends on the cause. If you have a low-grade fever with symptoms of cold or flu, home treatment with aspirin (provided you are not allergic) or acetaminophen taken every six hours may relieve muscle aches as well as lower your temperature. However, any drug treatment should be discussed with your doctor. Aspirin should not be used if your child has a fever since its use has been linked to a serious complication of certain viral illnesses called Reyes syndrome.

As part of the evaluation of any prolonged or unusual fever, your doctor will want to ask you if you have traveled recently, taken any drugs, or been exposed to any infections. After a careful physical examination, certain X-rays and laboratory tests may be necessary in order to make a diagnosis and prescribe appropriate treatment.

CALL YOUR DOCTOR WHEN:

- you have a prolonged low-grade fever (under 102 degrees Fahrenheit).
- your fever comes and goes over a period of weeks.

- you have a fever associated with neck stiffness, shaking chills, wet cough, convulsions, or severe headache (*call immediately*).
- you have an extremely high fever (over 103 degrees Fahrenheit) for 12-24 hours.

WEIGHT LOSS AND/OR LOSS OF APPETITE

DESCRIPTION

If you're losing weight very gradually and eating normally, chances are you won't notice any weight loss until a friend or family member tells you how thin you look. Or you may suddenly realize that your clothes are too large, your glasses seem to be sliding off your nose, or your dentures are loose. These are all signs of possible significant weight loss, and you should consult your physician about them. Marked weight loss can sometimes occur in the absence of serious physical illness, or it can be caused by a wide variety of acute or chronic diseases, including cancer, infection, and hormone disorders.

Loss of appetite (anorexia) can occur with or without weight loss. Typically, your appetite will decrease whenever you have an infection such as a cold or flu. The same may be true when you're feeling stressed. However, severe and prolonged loss of appetite suggests a more serious problem. Causes include hormone disorders, intestinal diseases, cancer, and depression. In these cases, medical attention is necessary.

A severe emotional illness resulting in significant weight loss is called anorexia nervosa (*see* Eating Disorders). This condition is most common in young women who have an intense fear of getting fat.

WHEN TO BE CONCERNED

You should always regard unintentional significant weight loss as a serious symptom. Consult your doctor. The same is true whenever you experience a loss of appetite that does not return quickly and can't be explained by some obvious cause such as a cold or flu.

TREATMENT

To treat weight loss and/or a decreased desire to eat, you must find and treat the underlying cause. Your doctor may need to do special tests, including X-rays, as part of his evaluation. If he determines that the cause is psychological, you may need counseling, with or without medication.

CALL YOUR DOCTOR WHEN:

- you notice significant weight loss despite eating normally.
- you experience loss of appetite in the absence of any mild underlying disease such as a cold.
- your loss of appetite lasts longer than one week.
- your loss of appetite is associated with severe depression.

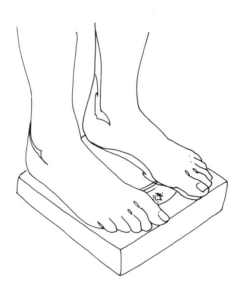

WEIGHT GAIN AND/OR SWELLING

DESCRIPTION

For many people, weight gain is a chronic problem, and large numbers of Americans are significantly overweight. Experts consider any individual who is 10 percent over ideal body weight to be obese.

For most people, a few extra pounds represent a cosmetic rather than a health problem. Whenever you eat more calories than you burn, you'll gain weight. Your excess intake may result from both physical and emotional factors. A change to a sedentary lifestyle, a move to a different climate, a sudden illness, or simply a change in your work may be the cause. Even if you're not eating more, you'll still notice a gradual weight gain.

More often, a recent change in your eating habits will be the cause of a gradual weight gain. You may have increased your food intake as a result of a recent emotional upset or a change in your social life. Regardless of the cause, remember that you must balance the number of calories you consume with the number of calories you burn in your normal daily activities. Each pound of body fat represents approximately 3,500 calories.

Generally, all calories you eat are the same, regardless of which foods supply them or when you eat them. But anxiously and compulsively counting calories is difficult and usually not very effective. Just remember that sudden changes in your diet or exercise will begin to affect your weight very quickly.

Although you may have read that exercise burns few calories, regular, vigorous exercise will significantly affect your weight. Some experts feel that regular exercise not only burns off calories but actually changes the way your body metabolizes fats and carbohydrates.

Attain your ideal weight without "crash" or "fad" diets. These diets may lead to rebound compulsive eating or to other eating disorders such as bulimia or anorexia nervosa (*see* Eating Disorders). It is now generally believed that a behavior modification program combined with regular exercise is the most effective way to lose weight and to keep it off.

First, it is important that you determine your ideal body weight. For anyone, being overweight presents a very clear health risk. If you have heart disease, high blood pressure, or diabetes, you are at an even higher risk for complications. In most of these cases, weight loss will markedly alleviate your symptoms.

Another less common cause of weight gain is fluid retention or a buildup of fluid in your body tissues (edema). You will most often notice this as a swelling around your feet, ankles, or calves. Fluid may also accumulate less obviously in your abdomen or in other tissues of your body. Fluid buildup in the feet and ankles is common in people who are on their feet all day. It also occurs frequently in people who wear tight undergarments such as garters or girdles. Women may experience some fluid retention prior to their menstrual periods. This should disappear when menstruation begins. Another common cause of fluid retention is the intake of excess salt.

WHEN TO BE CONCERNED

Edema is not a disease in itself, but it may be a symptom of serious underlying disease such as heart failure, liver disease, or kidney disease. Repeated episodes of swelling of your feet or ankles that last more than two or three days, unusual puffiness of your face, or swelling of your abdomen should be reported to your physician. If this swelling is also associated with any shortness of breath, seek *immediate* medical attention.

TREATMENT

If you have any significant weight gain, particularly if it is sudden, see your doctor. He'll do a complete evaluation to find the cause and prescribe proper treatment. If your problem is excess calorie intake, he will likely suggest a weight control program combined with behavior modification and exercise. If you are retaining fluid, he may advise you to restrict your salt intake in addition to other treatment.

CALL YOUR DOCTOR WHEN:

- you are more than 10 percent over your normal body weight.
- you notice a significant weight gain, especially if it is sudden.
- you have repeated episodes of swelling in your legs or ankles that last more than two or three days, unusual puffiness of your face, or swelling of your abdomen.
- swelling is associated with shortness of breath (*call immediately*).

ITCHING

DESCRIPTION

Itching is that unpleasant sensation in the skin that leads to a desire to scratch. You may also experience itching as a stinging, crawling, or burning feeling. These sensations arise when the nerve endings in the skin are stimulated. Many people find itching far less tolerable than pain.

So why are you itching? There are many possible reasons. Temporary, mild itching may be unrelated to any underlying problem and will just go away by itself. On the other hand, itching can be a symptom of certain infectious diseases such as measles or chicken pox (*see* Generalized Rashes). Even fungal infections like athlete's foot (*see* Athlete's Foot) may make you want to scratch. If you are allergic to certain foods, you may notice intense itching associated with a generalized rash that looks like red round wheals on your skin (hives). Poison ivy is another kind of allergy that makes you itch. Insect bites as well as infestation with certain parasites, like lice (*see* Lice) or itch mites (scabies) (*see* Scabies) are also associated with itching.

Perhaps the most common cause of generalized itching is excessive dryness of the skin. This is particularly true in elderly people. Sensitivity to drugs, soaps, or makeup can cause either generalized or localized itching.

Occasionally, itching without a visible cause can be triggered by underlying psychological stress. Often the itching will occur in varied areas such as your neck, forearms, or scalp. Removing the stress or learning to control it effectively usually stops the itching.

WHEN TO BE CONCERNED

Sometimes generalized itching is a warning that something more serious is going on. If there is no obvious underlying cause, such as an insect bite, exposure to poison ivy, or dry skin, your doctor will want to check you for certain underlying illnesses such as diabetes, thyroid disease, kidney failure, liver disease, or even cancer.

If you are taking medication and you experience itching, check with your doctor *immediately* to see if that's the cause. Ordinarily, you should not discontinue a drug without your doctor's advice unless you are having a severe reaction.

TREATMENT

Treatment of itching is usually aimed at treating or removing the underlying cause. Avoid things you know irritate your skin, such as rough clothing or certain makeup. If you have very dry or irritated skin, don't use detergents or harsh soaps. Skin lotions or cream may alleviate the dryness. You might want to take baths with a small amount of bath oil. Just remember, excessive bathing and soaking in water can also lead to dry skin. To avoid infection, keep your nails trimmed and clean and, if possible, don't scratch.

CALL YOUR DOCTOR WHEN:

- there is no underlying cause of your itching such as an insect bite or exposure to poison ivy.
- the itching persists for more than a week.
- the itching is associated with any other symptoms, such as rash, and you can't find the cause.
- you notice a general discoloration of your skin (jaundice) (*see* Jaundice).
- you are taking medication and develop itching (*call immediately*).

COUGH AND/OR SHORTNESS OF BREATH

DESCRIPTION

A cough is one way your body prevents irritating particles that enter your airways from invading your lungs. Viruses and bacteria that cause infection, as well as dust, smoke, and pollen, are trapped in the tiny hairs (cilia) that line your air passages and act as protective barriers. Irritation of these cilia stimulates your cough reflex.

Whenever you develop a cough, you should determine its cause. For example, a cough at work when inhaling certain noxious chemicals may indicate an allergy to these substances. A cough during pollen season may also suggest allergy. Sometimes drinking hot or cold liquids or getting food "down the wrong pipe" can irritate the sensitive airways and provoke a cough.

Whether your cough is "dry" or "wet" will also be a clue to its cause. A dry cough usually occurs when the reflex is triggered by irritants such as smoke or dust or by allergies. Certain infections such as a cold, measles, or flu also commonly cause a dry cough. This type of cough should go away when the infection clears up. If it doesn't, there may be another cause, and you should consult your physician.

A wet cough means that you are coughing up fluid. In this case, your cough is likely from an infection in your lungs such as bronchitis or pneumonia. Once bacteria get past the protective barrier in the airways and actually invade the lungs, your body produces large amounts of sticky fluid (mucus) as a defense measure. This fluid irritates the lungs, causing you to cough it out. If this mucus is green, yellow, or reddish-brown, you probably have a lung infection and should seek medical advice. Whenever you cough up bright red blood, see your doctor *immediately*.

If you are a smoker (especially if you've been smoking a pack a day or more for years), you may cough every morning. This "smoker's cough" could be a symptom of chronic bronchitis. Consult your physician. Heavy smokers are much more likely to develop lung infections because nicotine in cigarettes destroys the cilia in the airways, leaving nothing to prevent viruses and bacteria from entering the lungs.

Shortness of breath is a symptom that may occur with or without a cough. Sometimes it comes on so gradually that you notice it only during strenuous activity. Regardless of when it occurs, this symptom requires your doctor's *immediate* attention since it means that you are unable to get enough oxygen into your system. You may have a feeling of breathlessness. Shortness of breath can be a symptom of bronchitis, asthma, emphysema, cancer, or heart disease.

WHEN TO BE CONCERNED

Anytime you have a dry cough persisting for longer than a week without other symptoms of a cold or flu, seek a doctor's advice. A wet cough suggests a possible lung infection and may require treatment with antibiotics. Although a cough is the most common symptom of respiratory disease, it may also be caused by other problems, such as heart disease. Shortness of breath with or without a cough requires a doctor's immediate attention.

TREATMENT

Because coughing is an important defense mechanism, you should generally avoid suppressing it. This is especially true of a wet cough. Before taking any cough suppressant, check with your doctor. On the other hand, an expectorant will help you cough up the fluid and possibly shorten your illness. Expectorants are sold over the counter without a prescription.

If your cough persists or is associated with shortness of breath, have your doctor determine the cause and suggest appropriate treatment. As part of his evaluation, he may order X-rays, examine and culture the fluid, and/or perform special breathing tests. If you are a smoker, you can prevent most serious lung problems by quitting (*see* Positive Health Care, Part I).

CALL YOUR DOCTOR WHEN:

- your dry cough persists for longer than a week and is not associated with a cold or flu.
- you are coughing up green, yellow, or reddish-brown fluid.
- you cough up bright red blood (*call immediately*).
- you are a smoker and cough every day.
- you are short of breath with or without a cough (*call immediately*).

GENERALIZED BONE AND JOINT SWELLING AND PAIN

DESCRIPTION

Your skeleton is made up of approximately 200 separate bones. This complex system of bones, ligaments, and tendons literally helps to "keep you in shape." Your bones support your skin and muscles and also surround and protect your internal organs.

Most people don't realize that bone is actually living tissue. Any injury or infection of bone is usually quite painful. A bone may be bruised from any blunt injury. If severe, such bruises may take several weeks to heal. Persistent pain, localized in a particular bone or area of a bone, may also be a symptom of something more serious, such as a bone infection (osteomyelitis) or even a tumor in the bone.

Most people tend to confuse bone pain with joint pain. Generalized bone pain is often a vague symptom that accompanies viral infections such as the flu. You may also have a low-grade fever and muscle aches and pains.

Your joints are formed by the union of two or more bones. Most of your joints are supported by tough fibrous bands (ligaments) and enclosed in capsules (bursa) that protect and lubricate them. Localized joint pain is a symptom that usually follows an injury to a ligament or cartilage or an inflammation of a bursa (*see* Symptoms and Diseases Affecting the Bones, Joints, and Muscles). Another cause of localized joint pain is a condition called gout. If you have gout, you've probably had attacks before. The pain is usually localized in one joint, which is often red and swollen.

Generalized joint pain is usually not a serious symptom unless it persists for more than several days or comes and goes. Usually it is one symptom of a viral illness, along with fever and muscle aches. When joint pains do persist, they may be a symptom of a generalized infection, arthritis, or other serious illness.

WHEN TO BE CONCERNED

If you have localized bone pain that did not result from a bruise, and it persists for more than a week, see your doctor. When you also have symptoms of fever, weight loss, or redness and swelling over the bone, immediate care is required. Generalized bone pain that persists or is associated with fever and weight loss should also be reported to your doctor.

Sudden severe pain in a single joint following an injury or a strenuous activity should be checked. Review the section on Symptoms and Diseases Affecting the Bones, Joints, and Muscles in Part III. Sudden pain with redness and swelling (particularly in your big toe) should make you suspect gout. Your doctor will do special tests to confirm this diagnosis.

Generalized joint pain of a few days' duration as one symptom of a cold or flu is usually nothing to worry about. If it persists, suspect a form of arthritis or a more serious condition. Fever, chest pain, and shortness of breath associated with generalized joint pains likewise require prompt medical evaluation and treatment.

TREATMENT

Home treatment for a bruise consists of cold packs to relieve the swelling. Avoid further injury to a bruised area. If your doctor suspects an infection or a tumor, he will order X-rays to confirm his diagnosis. Bone infections may require hospitalization and intravenous antibiotics.

Localized joint pain due to trauma usually requires splinting of the injured joint. Avoid putting weight or further strain on the joint. Cold packs may help reduce swelling. Your doctor will check the injured joint and order X-rays if he suspects a fracture or dislocation. If your pain is severe, he may prescribe pain medication and possibly an anti-inflammatory drug. If your joint is infected or you have gout, your doctor will diagnose and treat the underlying disease.

For generalized joint pain associated with a viral illness like a cold or flu, aspirin (if you are not allergic) or acetaminophen, bed rest, and plenty of fluids should relieve your symptoms. *Do not give your child aspirin for any viral infection* (*see* Fever in Infants and Children).

If your joint pain persists for over a week or is intermittent, your doctor may need special tests to make the diagnosis.

CALL YOUR DOCTOR WHEN:

- you have pain localized in a particular bone.
- you have generalized bone pain lasting more than a week.
- you have either localized or generalized bone pain associated with fever, weight loss, or redness or swelling over any bone.
- you experience sudden joint pain associated with an injury.
- you have sudden joint pain with redness and swelling.
- you have generalized joint pain that lasts more than a week or recurs on a regular basis.

ABDOMINAL PAIN, NAUSEA, VOMITING, OR DIARRHEA

DESCRIPTION

While most people really don't even begin to understand the anatomy of their digestive systems, almost everyone has experienced abdominal pain, nausea, vomiting, or diarrhea at some time. When you think of your digestive system, you probably think only of your stomach. Actually, your digestive system really begins at your lips and ends at your rectum. In between, you have approximately 27 feet of intestine and many different tissues and organs that work together to digest your food.

In evaluating what seem to be digestive symptoms, your doctor must suspect diseases of other systems as well. For example, sometimes a heart attack may cause symptoms identical to heartburn or indigestion (*see* Heartburn/Indigestion). Similarly, a brain tumor can cause symptoms of nausea and vomiting. Because of these confusing patterns, it is especially important that you give your doctor a careful medical history when you are describing any of these symptoms so that he can get at the real cause of your problems.

If you have frequent, repeated, or lasting severe abdominal pain (*see* Abdominal Cramping and Distention), you should consult your doctor. Try to describe the onset of the pain. If it came on suddenly over several minutes, it is likely due to a perforated ulcer or a blockage in the blood supply to your intestine. If your pain came on gradually over several hours, a diagnosis of appendicitis, gallstones, or possibly even a pelvic infection are possibilities.

The character of your abdominal pain is also a clue to the underlying cause. Colic or spasm of a portion of your intestine is the most common cause of abdominal pain. This type of pain is usually caused by a blockage somewhere in your intestinal tract, which stretches the intestine behind the blockage. A burning or aching type of pain is more characteristic of an ulcer.

The location of your abdominal pain is likewise very important in helping to determine its cause. Pain caused by appendicitis, for example, almost always settles in your right lower abdomen. Pain from bleeding or infection in your abdomen usually is widespread. Remember, when you complain of abdominal pain, your stomach is not always where the pain really begins.

Other symptoms, such as nausea and vomiting (*see* Nausea and Vomiting), when associated with abdominal pain, may give your doctor further clues to your diagnosis. Although nausea and vomiting are usually not symptoms of a serious illness, they should not be taken lightly. Too, the first sign of pregnancy often will be the nausea and vomiting commonly known as "morning sickness."

Diarrhea is also a symptom that is usually not serious. The most common cause is probably a viral infection in your colon. However, the cause may also be bacterial. Although your colon normally contains a heavy growth of bacteria, a shift in the type, as occurs in "traveler's diarrhea" or following the use of antibiotics, can sometimes cause severe diarrhea. If your diarrhea persists or is associated with severe cramps, bloody stools, or fever and chills, get prompt medical attention. Your doctor's first question will almost always be "Have you traveled recently?"

If your symptoms are persistent and are associated with weight loss, your doctor will look for more serious causes. Be prepared to discuss your diet, the character of your stool, the amount of your weight loss, any medications you are taking, or any other medical problems that you have. It is important to realize that any change in your bowel habits (*see* Change in Bowel Habits) may be a very important symptom of a serious underlying condition.

WHEN TO BE CONCERNED

Any persistent abdominal pain, nausea, vomiting, or diarrhea can be a clue to a serious medical problem. These symptoms may not only suggest a problem with your digestive system, but they can also be a clue to other conditions as well. Remember that, whenever any of these symptoms are associated with intestinal bleeding, fever, chills, weight loss, or severe abdominal pain, you should seek medical evaluation as soon as possible.

TREATMENT

Only treat any of these symptoms at home when they are mild and of short duration. Generally, home treatment consists of avoiding any offending substance that you suspect has caused your nausea, vomiting, cramps, or diarrhea. Stay on a clear liquid diet until your symptoms go away in a day or two.

Your doctor will want to know how long you have had this symptom and how often you vomit. He'll ask about the character of your vomitus and many doctors will actually want to see a sample and possibly test it for blood or other substances.

Your doctor's treatment of more severe or prolonged symptoms will depend on his diagnosis of the underlying cause. Many very sophisticated diagnostic tools are now available that actually permit a specialist to look directly at large portions of your digestive system and diagnose any abnormalities. In addition to his direct observation, your doctor will have many other laboratory and X-ray studies available if he determines that they are necessary to find the cause of your symptoms.

CALL YOUR DOCTOR WHEN:

- you have any severe abdominal pain, nausea, vomiting, or diarrhea.
- you have any of these symptoms associated with bleeding, fever, chills, or weight loss (call immediately).

BLEEDING OR ABNORMAL BRUISING

DESCRIPTION

Everyone has had a cut, a nosebleed, or a tooth pulled. Whatever the reason, anytime a blood vessel is torn, blood leaks into the tissues. Usually, this bleeding stops within minutes. Certain substances (factors) in your blood together with special blood cells (platelets) react quickly to make your blood clot.

If any of these factors is missing, or if there is a problem with your platelets, your blood will not clot properly and you will continue to bleed even after minor injuries. In either case, bleeding may occur anywhere in your body with possible serious blood loss. Abnormal clotting, or lack of clotting, may be caused by malnutrition, infections, drug reactions, anemia, leukemia, or inherited disorders like hemophilia.

If your blood vessels are weakened or damaged for any reason, you may bruise easily. The bruises that some women notice on their thighs or hips called "devil's pinches" are usually not serious but should always be evaluated by a physician. Elderly people with very thin skin may also bruise easily, especially on the backs of their hands and on their forearms. This is usually not a cause for concern.

WHEN TO BE CONCERNED

Any abnormal bleeding should be a cause for concern. While bleeding is normal in women each month (menstruation), it is not normal between periods, and menstruation generally should not last longer than five to seven days or be extremely heavy. If it is, consult your physician. You may occasionally have a mild nosebleed or bleeding from your gums, but if the bleeding persists, is extremely heavy, or occurs frequently, call your doctor. Any blood in your urine, stool, vomitus, or sputum requires immediate medical attention. Easy bruising, especially if it is frequent and unrelated to any injury, must be checked. Likewise, see your physician if bruising is associated with other symptoms such as fever, joint pain and swelling, or abdominal pain.

TREATMENT

If you are bleeding heavily (hemorrhaging), the first step is obviously to stop the blood loss and determine the cause. If possible, apply direct pressure to the bleeding site. If the bleeding is from an arm or leg injury, you may use a tourniquet but loosen it every few minutes. If your gums are bleeding, try packing with cotton gauze temporarily. For nosebleeds, lean forward and pinch your nostrils. Never bend your head back; avoid swallowing the blood.

If your bleeding is caused by a clotting abnormality, you may need tests to determine the exact problem. Severe internal bleeding may require emergency surgery to prevent significant blood loss or damage to an organ. Know your blood type and carry adequate identification with you at all times in case you require an emergency blood transfusion.

CALL YOUR DOCTOR WHEN:

- you are bruising without any apparent reason.
- you notice bleeding that doesn't stop after a few minutes (*call immediately*).
- you have excessive or abnormal bleeding (*call immediately*).
- you have blood in your urine, stool, vomitus, or sputum (*call immediately*).

PART III

SYMPTOMS AND DISEASES AFFECTING SPECIFIC BODY SYSTEMS

Chapter 5

Symptoms and Diseases Affecting the Skin and Mucous Membranes

BALDNESS AND HAIR LOSS

DESCRIPTION

Many men worry about losing their hair. Typical male-pattern baldness (receding hairline) is extremely common and tends to run in families. Most people don't realize that this type of baldness can be inherited from either parent. In other words, if every man on your mother and father's side of the family had plenty of hair well into old age, you probably will too. Women can also become bald, but this loss is generally confined to thinning of the hair on the front and sides of the scalp. Women may notice some hair loss or thinning after pregnancy. Again, this will generally reverse itself without any treatment. Complete baldness is rare in women.

A sudden and usually temporary hair loss may follow certain illnesses (especially those associated with high fever), stressful periods, the use of certain drugs (particularly cancer-fighting agents), or overdoses of vitamin A.

51

WHEN TO BE CONCERNED

If you notice sudden hair loss on small areas on your scalp, eyebrows, or eyelashes (or, in men, your beard) or total loss of all hair, this may be a condition called alopecia areata or loss of hair in certain well-defined areas of the scalp. Your doctor will want to do a complete examination and certain laboratory tests to determine the cause.

TREATMENT

There is no known effective treatment for male-pattern baldness, but researchers are currently investigating a few promising new drugs. Some dermatologists and plastic surgeons have had some success with hair transplants.

If your hair loss is temporary, your doctor will need to evaluate and treat the underlying cause. If you have alopecia areata, depending on its severity, your doctor may prescribe steroid treatments. A wig can cover the bald areas and minimize concern over hair loss while undergoing therapy.

CALL YOUR DOCTOR WHEN:

- you have sudden hair loss on your scalp, eyebrows, eyelashes, or beard or total hair loss.
- you have male-pattern baldness and want to discuss available treatment.

DANDRUFF

DESCRIPTION

Nearly everybody seems to worry about dandruff, that itchy condition that plagues your scalp and sprinkles your clothes with small white flakes. It is so common that hair care manufacturers have made literally millions of dollars selling you their products. Actually, while dandruff may cause some embarrassment and discomfort, it is generally not serious.

Dandruff usually represents an increase in the normal loss of the outermost skin layer. The small flakes, which are actually dead skin, fall away when the hair is brushed or combed. Some types of dandruff are associated with inflammation of the scalp (seborrheic dermatitis), causing widespread yellow-red scaling to appear along the hairline, behind the ears, in the outer ear canal, on the eyebrows, on the bridge of the nose, in the area between the nose and mouth, and over the breastbone. Even this severe form, however, does not cause hair loss (*see* Baldness and Hair Loss). Both heredity and climate seem to determine whether you will have dandruff and how severe it will be. It is usually worse in winter.

WHEN TO BE CONCERNED

When you notice widespread scaling along your hairline, eyebrows, outer ears, near your nose and mouth, or on your chest, as described above, especially if there is associated crusting of your eyelids or eye irritation, your doctor will need to evaluate your condition in order to determine the best treatment. He will also need to make sure this is not another condition altogether, such as psoriasis or eczema.

TREATMENT

Treatment depends on the location and severity of the condition. For simple dandruff, a shampoo containing zinc pyrithione, selenium sulfide, or sulfur should be used every other day until your dandruff is controlled and twice a week thereafter. These shampoos

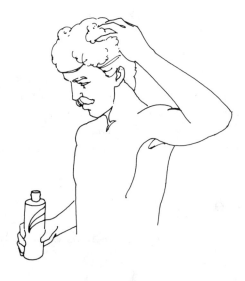

are sold in most pharmacies without a prescription. If your dandruff is more severe, your doctor may want to prescribe a stronger shampoo and/or a steroid preparation.

CALL YOUR DOCTOR WHEN:

- your dandruff becomes unmanageable.
- you notice widespread redness and scaling of the scalp.

EXCESS HAIR GROWTH

DESCRIPTION

Excess hair growth in areas of your body that are usually not hairy is known as hirsutism. Some women may experience it to varying degrees when reaching menopause because of the normal decrease in certain female hormones that prevent the growth of body hair. In younger women, men, and children, abnormal hormonal conditions may be the cause of excess hair growth. Occasionally, this is a side effect of taking certain drugs such as steroids or antidepressants.

WHEN TO BE CONCERNED

You should always consult your doctor when you notice excess hair growth.

TREATMENT

Treatment is aimed at determining and treating any underlying disorder, and for that you should consult your doctor. Plucking, shaving, and waxing to remove hair is generally a safe, but only temporary, solution. Chemical hair removers may irritate your skin. Before using these or trying electrolysis to destroy the individual hair follicles permanently, talk with your physician.

CALL YOUR DOCTOR WHEN:

- you notice excess hair growth in areas of your body usually not hairy.

GENERALIZED RASHES

DESCRIPTION

A generalized rash may be a symptom of a bewildering variety of different diseases, most of which are self-limited and harmless but a few of which may be serious. Usually, these rashes are caused either by infections such as measles, chicken pox, and roseola or by allergic reactions to such things as poison ivy, drugs, or foods. Generally, lice and scabies cause intense itching, but they do not cause a rash as such.

Most often, your rash will cause itching and burning, but sometimes it may be accompanied by other more serious symptoms, such as fever, cough, headache, or swollen glands. If you have a serious allergic reaction to a food or a drug, you may develop severe wheezing and shortness of breath in addition to hives.

If you develop a rash caused by an allergy to a food, drug, or chemical, it may be difficult for your doctor to determine the cause, so a comprehensive medical history is important. Try to recall any unusual foods or medications you have taken recently. Most allergic rashes look like typical hives, with large, red, raised patches of various sizes. Severe itching will usually be the primary symptom in allergic rashes.

Poison ivy is another type of allergen that causes a typical rash. Approximately 75 percent of people may be allergic to poison ivy. Although your first exposure may not produce the characteristic rash, a later exposure might. Typically, you'll soon develop a red, swollen, itchy rash with clusters of small and large blisters. Some cases can be quite serious, and the blisters can appear all over your body. You may be surprised to know that it is not contagious but rather an allergic reaction to a chemical in the leaves.

Measles is caused by a virus and is perhaps one of our most common childhood infections (*see* Fever in Infants and Children). If your child has measles, he or she will develop a typical rash three to five days after the onset of fever, cough, and cold symptoms. Brownish-pink spots will usually appear all over the body, with mild itching and characteristic whitish spots inside the mouth. Although these symptoms may suggest measles, you should consult your doctor to confirm the diagnosis.

Chicken pox is a viral illness, usually mild, with a very characteristic rash as well as other symptoms. It is most commonly a childhood disease (*see* Fever in Infants and Children) and is extremely contagious. The itching skin eruption begins as a spotty rash and gradually develops into raised teardrop-shaped blisters called vesicles. Eventually, these vesicles form scabs, which can easily become infected when they are scratched. If you get chicken pox as an adult, you will likely have a similar rash but with more severe symptoms and a higher risk of complications.

Lice and scabies are tiny parasites that may infect your skin and cause severe itching. Many people think that infestation is a sign of poor hygiene, but this is not necessarily true. You can readily get both of these infections from skin-to-skin contact or simply from the linens or clothes of a recently infested person. Lice more commonly make their home in the hairy portions of your body, while scabies are more common in the skin folds.

WHEN TO BE CONCERNED

A mild generalized rash, without other symptoms, that goes away when you have eliminated the cause usually does not require medical care. If your generalized rash persists longer than a week, or if you develop symptoms such as fever, chills, cough, headache, or swollen glands, see your doctor promptly.

Intense itching near the folds of your skin and a dark wavy line near the surface suggests scabies. If you actually see lice or their eggs (nits) in the hairy areas of your body, you should suspect lice as the cause of your itching. Often there is a secondary infection caused by repeated scratching.

If you experience the sudden onset of hives along with wheezing and shortness of breath, consider this an emergency requiring *immediate* medical attention.

TREATMENT

Most generalized rashes caused by infection are treated by treating the underlying disease. If your doctor suspects a bacterial infection, he may get cultures to help in his diagnosis and prescribe an appropriate antibiotic. Follow your doctor's advice carefully, because many of these infections can lead to serious complications.

Unfortunately, if your rash is caused by a viral illness such as measles or chicken pox, no medication will be effective. Your doctor will recommend isolation, plenty of rest, and increased fluids. Again, you must be careful to avoid other complications.

Lice and scabies require persistent and careful treatment to prevent recurrences. Kwell is a prescription medication commonly used to treat both parasites, and your doctor will give you careful instructions on its proper use. You will need to carefully clean all of your clothing, linens, and furniture, and generally other family members will also require treatment.

Treatment of most generalized rashes due to allergy involves removal of the offending substance. You can try saline compresses three times daily and calamine lotion locally to relieve the itching and swelling. If necessary, your doctor may prescribe antihistamines for added relief. More serious cases may require steroid medications applied topically to the skin or taken orally. If you have an acute allergic reaction with hives and severe shortness of breath, you should get to an emergency room *immediately*. In these cases, you may require oxygen, as well as intravenous fluids with steroids and adrenaline.

CALL YOUR DOCTOR WHEN:

- your generalized rash persists for longer than five to seven days, even without other symptoms.
- your generalized rash is associated with fever, chills, itching, cough, or headache.
- you have severe itching in the folds of your skin or you notice lice or their eggs in your hair.
- you experience a sudden outbreak of hives associated with wheezing or shortness of breath (*call immediately*).
- you are taking medication and develop a rash.

IRRITATION OF THE
MUCOUS MEMBRANES

DESCRIPTION

Mucous membranes are the moist membranes that line many of your body cavities, including your mouth, genitals, and rectum. These membranes may be the site of conditions such as canker sores, fever blisters, yeast infections, or even syphilis.

Those painful tiny white or red ulcers you get inside your cheeks, on your tongue, on your gums, or on your lips from time to time are very likely canker sores (aphthous ulcers). No one knows their exact cause. An iron, vitamin B_{12}, or folic acid deficiency may be a factor. Similarly, stress, certain foods, or even poorly fitting dentures may be a cause. Although they tend to recur, canker sores generally last no more than 7–10 days and go away without treatment. Usually, only the sores are painful, although you may also experience fever, fatigue, or swollen glands.

Fever blisters, or cold sores, affect 85 percent of the population at one time or another, often for the first time during infancy or childhood. The sores are caused by the herpes simplex type I virus. Once you have been exposed to the virus, it remains dormant in your body for years and may suddenly reappear as a sore on your lip, in your mouth, or near your nostrils. Stress, sun exposure, or even menstruation may cause reappearances. Once the blister develops, it opens within a few days, forming a yellowish crust that disappears within about 10 days. (The related herpes simplex type II virus is the cause of genital herpes and is discussed in the sections on Penile Pain and Vaginal Pain.)

If you have children, you may already know all about thrush. That's because this infection of the mouth, caused by the yeast Candida albicans, is fairly common in infants, especially if they are bottle-fed. Typically, your baby's tongue, throat, gums, or cheeks show white patches that look like milk curds. Because of mouth irritation, your baby may refuse feedings. Your doctor will recommend treatment. When this infection develops in older children or adults, it could be more serious.

A sore on your mucous membranes also may be syphilis. Syphilis is a sexually transmitted infection spread from person to person via intimate physical contact with infected parts of the body such as the genitals, rectum, or mouth.

The first sign of this infection (the primary phase) is usually a small, painless sore (chancre). Because it is painless, you may not notice it. Although this chancre is usually on the genitals, it may appear on your lips, tongue, rectum, or other mucous membranes. Even without treatment, the sore usually goes away in a few weeks, but your body still harbors the disease.

The second stage appears two to six months after you've been exposed. Symptoms include a non-itchy body rash (usually on the palms of your hands or the soles of your feet), sore throat, swollen glands, and sores in your mouth.

It may take four to six years after the first contact for tertiary or final stage syphilis to appear. Heart disease, blindness, skin lesions, and paralysis are possible symptoms.

WHEN TO BE CONCERNED

Canker sores are nothing to worry about. Except in babies and young children, herpes and canker sores may look very different. Herpes generally begins as a papule (a small white bump), then becomes a vesicle (blister), and then ruptures, at which point it may look very similar to a canker sore. Canker sores rarely appear on the front part of the roof of your mouth (your hard palate). Painless sores in your mouth or on your lips could be another, more serious condition such as syphilis and should be evaluated by your doctor. Whenever a painful sore doesn't go away within a week, consult your doctor.

Because fever blisters also go away without treatment, you generally don't need to be concerned about them. There are complications that can be quite serious, however, such as eye infections. If you have a fever blister and also have irritation or pain in your eye, call your doctor immediately. Do the same if you have an illness such as eczema or are taking steroids internally.

If you've been taking antibiotics for a long time, you may develop thrush as a side effect of the treatment. Sometimes, however, thrush in older children and adults may be a clue to a more serious condition.

TREATMENT

Because canker sores go away on their own, they don't require treatment. Avoid certain foods that seem to bring them on. If they are very painful, you can purchase carbamide peroxide in glycerol (Gly-Oxide) or benzocaine (Orajel or Anbesol) at any pharmacy. Follow the directions. Avoid eating salty or acidic foods. Never use a steroid cream (Cortaid, for example) without first checking with your doctor.

There is no cure for oral herpes simplex. You can often prevent these by using a sunscreen when you sunbathe. If you already have a fever blister, petroleum jelly (e.g., Vaseline) and certain compounds containing phenol (such as Blistex) may relieve your pain. Good nutrition and rest may help to speed your recovery. Because fever blisters are highly contagious, avoid kissing anyone until the sores completely disappear. Avoid spreading the virus to your eyes or other parts of your body by washing your hands carefully if you happen to touch the blisters.

Thrush is generally treated with a medication called Nystatin. This is available only by prescription, and your doctor will instruct you on how to use it.

Antibiotics are used to treat syphilis. Proper treatment in the early stages completely cures the disease. Avoid intimate contact with anyone who has the disease. If you have several sexual partners, get a blood test for syphilis regularly.

CALL YOUR DOCTOR WHEN:

- you have painful sores on your hard palate.
- you have sores in your mouth that don't disappear in a week.
- you have a painless sore on your mucous membranes.
- your infant or young child has painful sores in his mouth or on his lips, especially if there is associated fever or swollen glands (this could be herpes).
- you have eczema or are taking steroids internally and develop a fever blister.
- your eye becomes irritated and/or painful and you have a fever blister (*call immediately*).
- you notice white curdlike patches in your mouth or throat.
- you have had intimate contact with someone who has syphilis.

OTHER SKIN IRRITATIONS: ACNE AND BOILS

DESCRIPTION

Acne (acne vulgaris) is the most common of all skin conditions. It generally begins in your teenage years when your body starts producing certain hormones (androgens) that increase the size and activity of glands in your skin (sebaceous glands). The oily substance these glands produce (sebum) cannot escape when your hair follicles become blocked by a plug made of protein (keratin). When this plug turns black, a blackhead is formed. Acne occurs mainly on the face, neck, upper chest, back, and shoulders. Besides pimples, you may notice mild soreness, pain, or itching of your skin. Self-consciousness and embarrassment are probably the most disturbing effects, even though acne is almost universal.

Any localized collection of pus in your body is called an abscess. An abscess forms when the pus becomes surrounded and walled off by the damaged tissues. When this occurs under your skin, it may become very tender and it is called a boil. Boils will occur most frequently on your neck, breast, face, and buttocks. They will tend to be especially painful when they occur in small anatomical areas such as your nose, ears, or fingers. Boils are usually red, raised, and swollen, and they eventually rupture, allowing the pus to drain. In spite of general good health and careful hygiene, you should not be alarmed if you occasionally develop a boil.

A carbuncle is generally a cause for more concern. This is usually a collection of boils. The carbuncle drains through many channels called sinuses underneath the skin. Although carbuncles develop more slowly than a single boil, they will often be associated with fever, chills, and weakness. These more serious skin infections usually occur in men and most commonly on the back of the neck.

WHEN TO BE CONCERNED

Although acne is usually mild, contrary to popular belief, it does not always disappear when you become an adult. In some cases, acne can become severe and chronic, causing infected cysts and scarring of your skin. That is when treatment by a physician becomes important.

If you develop a boil that is especially large, painful, or associated with fever, you should consult your doctor. Boils located in the nose or ear or near the eye also require prompt medical attention. Frequent or multiple boils, or boils that do not drain and heal promptly, may signal a more serious underlying illness. For example, diabetics or individuals with other debilitating diseases will often suffer from frequent skin infections.

TREATMENT

Despite what you may have heard, diet has little effect on acne. You can help the course of this condition, however, by washing several times a day with any mild toilet soap, especially if your face is oily. Avoid topical steroid creams or ointments since these may actually worsen your acne. If your acne is severe, your doctor may want to treat you with oral antibiotics or one of several drugs approved by the FDA for acne.

Although anyone may develop an occasional boil, it is important to begin treatment as soon as possible. Intermittent, hot compresses applied every two or three hours will usually cause the boil to come to the surface and drain spontaneously. These compresses should be continued once drainage begins. Keep the drainage site covered with sterile gauze as it heals.

Remember that boils on the neck or face or boils elsewhere that do not drain and heal promptly may require your doctor to prescribe oral antibiotics. If possible, he will culture the drainage to determine the type of infection so that an effective antibiotic can be prescribed. Infections in these areas that go untreated can seriously damage the underlying tissues. In more serious cases, your doctor may recommend intravenous antibiotics and surgical drainage of the pus.

CALL YOUR DOCTOR WHEN:

- your acne appears severe and/or chronic.
- starting any antibiotic therapy.
- a single boil is located in the nose or ear or near the eye.
- a single boil does not begin to drain and heal in three to four days with hot compresses.

- a single boil is especially large, painful, or associated with fever and/or chills.
- a single boil keeps recurring.
- you have multiple boils or carbuncles.
- you have an underlying medical problem such as diabetes.

SKIN DISCOLORATIONS

DESCRIPTION

Birthmarks are just that—pink, red, or purplish marks anywhere on your skin that are usually present when you are born. Some birthmarks appear shortly after birth. As many as one-third of all newborns have birthmarks. Most go away by themselves by age six. If you have a birthmark and are an adult, the worst problem for you is probably cosmetic.

Almost all of us have a few moles. They are areas of pigment in your skin and can occur anywhere on the body. Moles can be flesh-colored or differently pigmented. They can be large or small, flat or raised, smooth, hairy, or warty in appearance. If you have any moles, they probably first appeared when you were a child or teenager. Pregnant women normally seem to get more moles during pregnancy, and the moles that they already have may become larger and darker.

A wart is a noncancerous skin growth caused by a virus. Plantar warts are those that appear on the soles of your feet, usually at the base of your toes.

The black-and-blue marks you get on your skin when you bump yourself are called bruises (*see* Bleeding or Abnormal Bruising). After an injury, blood escapes from the small vessels just beneath your skin. First the color is red or pink, then bluish-black, then greenish-yellow as it fades and resolves. Occasional bruising is not ordinarily significant.

Some people always look pale, especially if they are fair-skinned or don't go out in the sun very often. However, true pallor is generally caused by reduced blood flow to the skin and other organs. It may be a sign of something quite serious such as anemia or heart disease.

Just before you faint, you may notice pallor (*see* Dizziness, Vertigo, or Loss of Consciousness).

Since it is often hard to detect pallor in the skin, especially if it develops gradually, you should look at the inner part of your lower eyelid, your lips, the inside of your mouth, or the skin under your fingernails. If these places seem unusually pale, it is possible that you have pallor.

Most people think of jaundice as a yellowish discoloration of the skin and eyes. It often appears gradually and isn't noticed until other symptoms such as nausea, vomiting, fever, "tea-colored" urine, chills, and fatigue develop. All causes of jaundice can be serious and require immediate medical care.

WHEN TO BE CONCERNED

Rarely, certain birthmarks may be a clue to more serious problems. These tend to be located over the face, especially the eye. If your baby has a birthmark, point it out to your doctor at your first well-baby checkup.

Most moles are nothing to worry about. However, some can become malignant and should be treated. If you have a mole that suddenly changes in size or color or begins to bleed, hurt, or itch, seek immediate medical advice.

Except for pain, you really don't need to worry about plantar warts. It's not unusual for them to disappear completely without any treatment.

If you bruise easily for no apparent reason and without any history of direct injury, you should get a medical evaluation. A tendency to develop several bruises at once, especially when they are larger than usual, is also a clue to abnormal clotting. Blackened stools, bleeding gums, or blood in your urine are additional symptoms of abnormal bleeding that require immediate medical attention. Likewise, if your bruising is associated with any fever, joint swelling or pain, abdominal pain, or shortness of breath, suspect a serious medical problem.

If you think you have pallor, especially if you have other associated symptoms such as fatigue or shortness of breath, contact your physician promptly.

If you notice that you are jaundiced or have a yellowish cast to your skin, see your doctor.

TREATMENT

Since most types of birthmarks go away on their own, no treatment is necessary. Some birthmarks that persist in adulthood can be treated surgically or with lasers, but you should follow your doctor's advice. If you are worried about the appearance of your birthmark, ask a cosmetic expert to prepare a cream to match your skin color and cover the mark.

Moles that change in color and grow rapidly should always be removed surgically. If you have a mole located in an area of irritation such as under your breasts or under your arms, your doctor may feel it should also be removed.

Small plantar warts need not be treated. If you have a large wart or a particularly painful one, consult your doctor. Plantar warts must be treated with care to prevent lasting painful scars. Freezing with liquid nitrogen, salicylic acid plaster, and/or cautery are examples of treatments used today. If the wart is on a weight-bearing area, ask your pharmacist for a metatarsal bar or foam pad. Place this under the wart to relieve pressure.

Occasional, isolated small bruises are usually not significant. If they are tender, you may treat them at home with cold packs. If you bruise easily and develop any of the other symptoms mentioned above, you will require a thorough medical evaluation to determine the underlying cause. Your doctor will treat you based on his diagnosis of your condition.

The treatment of both pallor and jaundice is aimed at diagnosing and treating the underlying condition. Your doctor will probably do some blood tests as well as a complete examination as part of his evaluation.

CALL YOUR DOCTOR WHEN:

- your child has a birthmark over the face, especially near the eye.
- you have a mole that suddenly gets bigger, turns darker in color (dark brown or black), begins to bleed, or becomes painful, irritated, or itchy.
- you have a mole in an area of irritation.
- you have a large and/or painful plantar wart that you want removed.

- you have bruises without any apparent cause.
- you have several bruises or very large bruises.
- your bruising is associated with other symptoms such as fever, joint pain and swelling, or abdominal pain.
- your skin appears yellow, regardless of other symptoms (*call immediately*).
- you notice unusual paleness of your skin, the inner part of your lower eyelids, the inside of your mouth, or your nailbeds, especially if there is associated fatigue or shortness of breath (*call immediately*).

Chapter 6

Symptoms and Diseases Affecting the Bones, Joints, and Muscles

NECK PAIN AND SYMPTOMS

DESCRIPTION

Usually, neck stiffness is a symptom that will cause you only mild discomfort. This stiffness or muscle cramping may be caused by a chill, by lying or sleeping in a cramped position, or by a sudden strain of the neck while driving or during strenuous sports. More severe spasm of the neck muscles is called torticollis.

"Whiplash" is a neck injury, commonly occurring as a result of an auto accident when you are hit from the rear. When this occurs, your neck is snapped backward and then forward. This can result in a strain or tear of the muscles or ligaments supporting your neck vertebrae. Although you may not develop pain for several hours, this is generally a more serious injury than a mild muscle spasm. Any movement of your neck may be extremely painful, and the pain may also radiate into your hands, with associated numbness or tingling.

A third common cause of neck pain is swelling of the glands in your neck (lymph nodes). Any infection of your head or neck, such as an abscess or a severe sore throat, can cause this. With severe

67

infections, these glands may get very large and tender so that just moving your neck may be quite painful.

In infants, a stiff neck may also be caused by an abscess behind the tonsil or, in very rare cases, by diphtheria. A stiff neck associated with a severe headache and fever can be a symptom of meningitis. This life-threatening emergency is due to an infection of the lining surrounding the brain and spinal cord.

Your thyroid gland is located in the front of your neck below your Adam's apple. Occasionally, this may become enlarged but rarely becomes tender. Your thyroid gland may also become enlarged when it is overactive.

WHEN TO BE CONCERNED

If you have neck pain caused by muscle spasms, you can usually relieve these symptoms in two or three days with simple home remedies such as hot compresses, whirlpool baths, massage, and, if necessary, two aspirin tablets three or four times a day (provided you're not allergic and don't have ulcer disease). You should seek medical advice when you have stiffness in your neck muscles without any apparent cause that is not relieved in two or three days with heat and aspirin. If there is also headache, fever, or lethargy along with neck stiffness or pain, see your doctor immediately.

Also seek medical attention if you have sudden neck trauma from a whiplash injury or a fall, especially if you experience any numbness or tingling in your hands or fingers. Any swelling in your neck, whether or not it is associated with pain or neck stiffness, should always be evaluated by your physician.

TREATMENT

If the stiffness or pain in your neck resulting from mild muscle spasm is not relieved with your home remedies, your physician may X-ray your neck to be certain that there is no serious underlying disorder. If he finds that your symptoms are due only to muscle strain, he may prescribe a muscle relaxant to relieve your spasm. If necessary, he may inject a local anesthetic into the tender areas of your neck muscles. Your doctor may also recommend physical therapy and neck exercises to strengthen the muscles.

If you have a whiplash-type injury that is severe, your doctor may request X-rays to be sure your vertebrae have not been injured. If you are in pain, he may prescribe muscle relaxants and pain medication along with a padded collar to support your neck muscles. In very severe cases, some form of traction may be necessary.

If your neck stiffness is due to swollen glands, it is important to diagnose and treat the underlying cause. If the cause is an abscess or another infection, antibiotics and drainage may be required. In rare cases, when neck stiffness is associated with severe headache, fever, or lethargy, your doctor may suggest a spinal tap to rule out meningitis. This severe infection requires *immediate* medical attention. If you experience neck swelling due to an enlarged thyroid, the underlying thyroid illness will need to be diagnosed and treated.

CALL YOUR DOCTOR WHEN:

- you have neck pain or stiffness persisting longer than two or three days that is unrelieved by hot compresses and aspirin.
- you have any neck stiffness associated with severe headache, fever, or lethargy (*call immediately*).
- you have neck pain and any numbness or tingling in your hands or fingers.
- you have any swelling or tenderness in the glands of your neck.
- you have neck pain or stiffness following an auto accident or other trauma (*call immediately*).
- you have any swelling or tenderness over the area of your thyroid.

NECK EXERCISES TO RELIEVE PAIN CAUSED BY STRESS

Stress can turn a figurative "pain in the neck" situation into a real physical neck pain and restricted neck motion, but stretching exercises can often help restore motion and relieve pain associated with stress. For maximum benefit, do these exercises in the shower or after applying hot, moist towels to increase blood flow to the muscles. Do the number of repetitions that are comfortable for you, but always stop when you begin to feel tired or feel increased pain. Do the exercises throughout the day to help relax and relieve tension of the neck and shoulder muscles.

Exercises

1. Stand up straight. Turn your head slowly as far as possible to the right. Return to normal center position and relax. Turn your head slowly as far as possible to the left. Return to normal center position and relax.

2. Stand up straight. Slowly lower your head and try to touch your chin to your chest. Slowly raise your head backward, looking up at the ceiling. Return to normal position and relax.

3. Stand up straight. Try to touch your left ear to the left shoulder. Return to normal center position and relax. Try to touch your right ear to the right shoulder. Return to normal center position and relax.

4. Stand up straight. Raise both shoulders as close to the ears as possible and hold. Count to five. Relax. Stretch your shoulders backward as far as possible and hold, then relax.

5. Stand up straight. With one hand, hold onto the thumb of the other hand behind the back, then pull downward toward the floor. Take a deep breath, stand on your toes, and look at the ceiling while exerting the downward pull. Hold for a few moments. Then exhale slowly and relax.

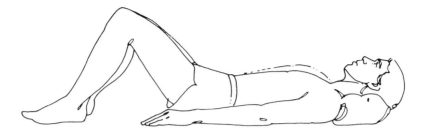

6. Lie on your back, knees bent, with a small pillow under your neck. Take a deep breath slowly, fully expanding chest, then exhale slowly. Repeat 10 times.

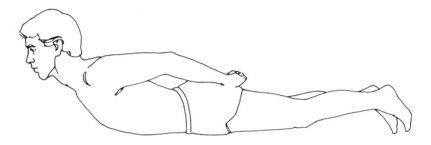

7. Lie on your stomach with your hands clasped behind your back. Pull your shoulders back and up by pushing your hands toward your feet, pinching shoulder blades together, and lift head from floor. Take a deep breath. Hold for two seconds. Relax. Repeat 10 times, both morning and night.

SHOULDER PAIN AND SYMPTOMS

DESCRIPTION

Shoulder pain has several possible causes. Your pain may develop gradually, without any clear cause, or suddenly, following a strenuous activity. This pain can be extremely disabling and in some cases may persist for months.

When your pain occurs suddenly, especially following a fall or other injury, it may be caused by a dislocation. If the ligaments supporting your shoulder are extremely weak, a dislocation can occur following any simple activity such as rolling over in bed or removing your coat. A few people tend to have repeated dislocations caused by certain vigorous activities such as swimming, tennis, or gymnastics. Usually, dislocations are extremely painful, but sometimes they may be only mildly uncomfortable or even painless.

If your shoulder pain came on gradually and became more severe over several days or weeks, suspect an inflammation known as bursitis. The bursa is a fluid-filled sac that lubricates the shoulder joint, and any injury or repeated stress can cause bursitis. Often, this chronic inflammation leads to a calcium deposit that causes pain in the tendon that raises your arm.

If your bursitis persists, or if you strained or tore the ligaments during a shoulder dislocation, you may develop a "frozen shoulder." This occurs when scar tissue forms in the joint and stiffens your shoulder, causing deep pain that may travel to your back, chest, or down your arm. As in many cases of muscle and bone pain, this may be worse at night.

WHEN TO BE CONCERNED

Suspect a shoulder dislocation when you have sudden pain and/or decreased motion after vigorous activity or after falling on your arm or shoulder. Carefully observe your injured shoulder in the mirror. If it has changed shape compared to your normal shoulder, see your doctor immediately. If your shoulder looks normal, but you still can't move it, or if you have numbness in your arm or hand, it may still be dislocated. Avoid moving your arm or trying to relocate the shoulder since this may injure the nerves and tendons.

If your shoulder pain began gradually, and you suspect bursitis, your shoulder should still look normal. The pain will occur mainly when you try to move it. If it has been injured for some time from a strain or tear of the tendons, or as the result of bursitis, it may have become stiff and painful. Consult your doctor so that he can diagnose and begin to treat your problem.

TREATMENT

After a sudden pain or trauma, if your doctor suspects a dislocation, an X-ray will confirm his diagnosis. He will attempt to relocate the shoulder, under anesthesia if necessary, as soon as possible to prevent damage to the nerves or tendons. He will likely immobilize your shoulder but suggest that you exercise your wrist and fingers. Follow his advice carefully to prevent permanent nerve and tendon damage and to be certain that you will not be prone to future dislocations.

If your shoulder pain follows a particularly strenuous activity, such as a weekend of house painting, you might assume that you have developed acute bursitis. Stop the activity and try (if you have no allergy or contraindication) two aspirin tablets three or four times a day along with cold packs to your shoulder. You may place your arm in a sling. In many cases, these home remedies will relieve your bursitis symptoms.

What if your pain persists? Your doctor may recommend treatment with steroids or other anti-inflammatory drugs. Usually, any calcium deposits that have formed will be absorbed in one to two weeks. Severe cases may require injecting a steroid and an anesthetic directly into your shoulder joint. Rarely, surgical removal of a calcium deposit will be necessary.

Once you've developed a "frozen shoulder," home remedies alone are usually not helpful. Your physician may suggest injecting an anesthetic into the shoulder, external heat, and ultrasound treatments. Physical therapy may also help relieve the stiffness, and special exercises will increase your range of motion (*see* illustration of shoulder exercises). Most cases of "frozen shoulder" will improve within six months to a year, but you may require prolonged physical therapy and exercises.

CALL YOUR DOCTOR WHEN:

- you experience a sudden loss of motion and/or pain in your shoulder following a strenuous activity or a fall.
- your affected shoulder looks different anatomically compared to your normal shoulder.
- your shoulder pain travels to your arm or hand or is associated with numbness or tingling (*call immediately*).
- your shoulder pain and stiffness came on gradually and are not relieved by aspirin, cold packs, and a sling.

EXERCISES FOR SHOULDER DISORDERS

General Instructions

Exercise is an excellent way to relieve stiffness and discomfort in your shoulder area. For maximum benefit, do these exercises after a shower or following application of hot, moist towels. Moist heat relieves pain by increasing blood flow to the muscles of your shoulders. As your condition gets better, gradually increase the number of times you repeat each exercise. As your pain tolerance increases, you will be able to increase the intensity and duration of these exercises. Repeat them two or three times a day to help relax and relieve tension of the shoulder muscles. Always stop when you begin to feel tired.

General Exercises

1. Stand up straight. Slowly raise your arms over your head. Stretch them as far as possible, keeping your elbows straight. Repeat and try to exceed the previous limit each time.

2. Stand up straight with your hands at your sides. Raise your arms laterally away from your sides. Bring them over your head and then clap your hands together, keeping your elbows straight. Repeat this exercise, bringing the backs of your hands together.

3. Stand up straight. With your hands locked behind your neck, pull your elbows backward and throw your chest outward as you extend your shoulders backward.

Continued on pages 76 and 77

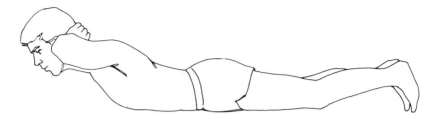

4. Lie on your stomach on a firm surface. With both hands at the back of your neck, raise your head and both elbows up from this surface. Do not raise your chest or the rest of your body.

5. Stand up straight. Place the back of the hand on the affected side on your lower back. Gradually try to move the hand up the back toward the opposite shoulder. If just one shoulder is affected, try to reach the same point on your back with the affected shoulder as you could with the normal shoulder. Repeat this exercise with the opposite hand if you are experiencing discomfort in both shoulders.

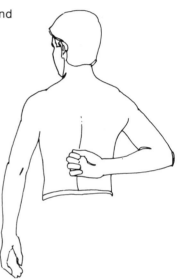

Wall-Climbing Exercise

Do this exercise for a total of approximately 15 minutes. Repeat two or three times a day.

1. Stand sideways, body straight, with your affected side to the wall. While keeping your elbow straight, walk your fingers up the wall and make a mark. Repeat this exercise 10 times, trying to exceed your previous mark each time.

2. Repeat the same procedure while facing the wall.

Pendulum Exercise

Do this exercise for approximately three minutes, two or three times a day. Your arm should swing free like a pendulum during the exercise. *Avoid overusing the affected shoulder.*

1. Lean forward and hold on to a table with the hand on the side of the *unaffected* shoulder. Hold a one- to two-pound weight in the hand on the *affected* side. With your shoulder relaxed, let your arm hang loosely. Swing arm forward and backward, keeping your elbow completely straight.

2. Next, keeping the weight in your hand, swing your arm laterally across your body, to the right and left. Keep your elbow straight.

3. Begin to make circles with your arm, beginning with small circles and gradually increasing the size of the circles.

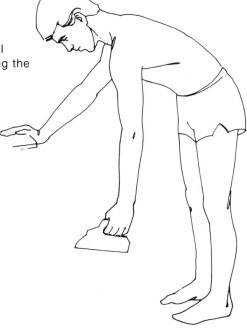

ELBOW PAIN AND SYMPTOMS

DESCRIPTION

"Tennis elbow" is the most common type of elbow pain, but it isn't necessarily caused only by playing tennis. Anytime you overuse the muscles of your forearm, the tendon at the outer border of your elbow can become inflamed. Using a screwdriver, clipping the garden hedge, or even lifting a cup of coffee may bring on the symptoms.

Like your shoulder joint, there is also a bursa (fluid-filled sac) surrounding your elbow joint. When the elbow bursa becomes irritated from an injury or because a piece of calcium is inside, pain, redness, and swelling behind your elbow joint develops (olecranon bursitis). Your elbow also may feel spongy.

WHEN TO BE CONCERNED

If the onset of your elbow pain is gradual following a particular activity or sport, and there is no history of a fall or other injury, you may wait a few days before seeking medical care. Compare your painful elbow to your other one to be sure there is no swelling or other deformity. You should be able to fully move your elbow slowly despite your pain.

When your pain occurs suddenly and is the result of a fall or other injury to the elbow, there may be a different type of bone injury, such as a fracture or dislocation. You may be unable to move your elbow joint because of this, and your pain may be severe. In this case, you should make a sling with a towel and safety pin to support your elbow and see your doctor as soon as possible. He will determine whether your injury is only tendinitis or bursitis rather than a fracture or dislocation of the elbow joint.

Also, you should be concerned if you experience any weakness, numbness, or more than momentary tingling in your forearm, hand, or fingers since they may indicate some damage to the nerve that runs over the elbow. Any irritation of this nerve (ulnar nerve) causes an electric-shock-like feeling in your hand and fingers. This is why the elbow is often known as the "crazy bone." Hand weakness may come on gradually. You may find that you have difficulty holding a book or a cup of coffee. Any of these symptoms may indicate nerve damage and should be evaluated promptly by your physician.

TREATMENT

If your pain has come on gradually following a particular irritating activity, you might try home treatment before seeking medical attention. Use a sling to keep the elbow from moving and apply cold packs every three or four hours. You may also take two aspirin tablets three or four times a day (if you are not allergic).

If your symptoms do not improve within four to five days, seek medical evaluation. If your doctor diagnoses tendinitis or bursitis, he may advise you to keep the elbow in a sling for a longer time and possibly prescribe steroids and other stronger drugs to decrease the inflammation. If the bursa is very swollen, your doctor may insert a needle and remove some of this fluid.

In severe cases, where a large calcium deposit develops in the elbow and does not go away by itself, surgical removal may be necessary. An X-ray will enable your doctor to evaluate a calcium deposit and also be certain that there is no fracture or dislocation of the elbow joint, especially if your pain has occurred after a fall or other injury. Finally, your doctor may consider injecting steroids directly into the bursa if the inflammation persists.

CALL YOUR DOCTOR WHEN:

- you have had a fall or other injury and are suddenly unable to move your elbow.
- you experience weakness, numbness, or continued tingling in your forearm, hand, or fingers.
- you notice a large swelling over your elbow.
- you have pain that has begun gradually after a particular activity and persists for more than four or five days despite home treatment.

WRIST PAIN AND SYMPTOMS

DESCRIPTION

Your wrist is a very complex anatomical structure that contains several small bones and ligaments. These connect the bones of your hand with the bones of your forearm. Your small wrist bones are perfectly positioned so that your wrist can normally move freely. The nerves to your fingers (see Hand Pain and Symptoms) pass through your wrist to direct the precise movements of your fingers.

The most common injury to the wrist is a sprain. This may occur while playing tennis or while using a heavy power tool. Although a simple wrist sprain can be quite painful, it usually is not serious, and there are usually no complications.

On the other hand, a dislocation or even a chip fracture of the small bones of your wrist can lead to serious complications if it is not diagnosed and treated promptly. Such delay can result in permanent stiffness of your wrist as well as damage to the nerves that control the sensation and strength in your hand and fingers.

Another common condition that is not serious is a small cystic growth on the wrist called a ganglion. This typically painless nodule appears on the back of your wrist out of the blue and often goes away by itself, sometimes after months. These cysts may be firm and as small as a pea. A ganglion usually contains fluid and rarely causes any problems.

WHEN TO BE CONCERNED

If your wrist pain has come on gradually, following a particular activity, try to be sure that it is only a sprain. Don't mistake a dislocation or small fracture for a simple sprain and delay getting treatment. Is there any weakness, numbness, or tingling in your fingers? Does your painful wrist look swollen or deformed compared with your normal wrist? If none of these other symptoms are present, you can try a course of home treatment.

When you suddenly injure your wrist by falling on your out-stretched hand, or when you severely sprain it, carefully evaluate your symptoms. Compare your injured wrist to your normal wrist. If it appears markedly swollen or deformed in any way, assume that it may be dislocated and see your doctor promptly. Delay in treating a dislocation or fracture of the wrist can result in poor healing of the injured small bones and permanent stiffness. Also, if you experience any weakness, numbness, or tingling in your hands or fingers, even in the absence of any apparent deformity of your wrist, see your doctor immediately.

If you have a persistent growth on your wrist, whether it is painful or not, you probably should have it checked by your doctor. If necessary, he will request an X-ray to help in his diagnosis.

TREATMENT

If you suspect that your sprain is mild, and if it did not result from a sudden injury but rather from a repeated strenuous activity such as using a power tool, you may try home treatment for a few days. Purchase a Velcro splint at your pharmacy to support your wrist and use cold packs and aspirin (if you're not allergic) for two or three days.

If your symptoms persist, see your doctor. He may advise an X-ray to be certain that you have not injured the bones of your wrist. Once your X-ray is negative, he may recommend a stronger anti-inflammatory medication or other treatment.

A fall or other sudden injury will be the most common cause of a wrist fracture or dislocation. Your doctor will order X-rays to determine the precise injury, and he will reset the fracture or dislocation. He will use a splint or a cast to keep the bones in position so that they heal properly. He will also try to prevent any permanent damage to the nerves or tendons of your hand.

Treatment of a ganglion cyst usually involves mere patience. Often, these small growths simply go away by themselves. If you have a small nodule on your wrist that persists for more than two months or becomes bothersome, your physician may consider removing the fluid with a small needle and injecting a steroid into the cyst. Rarely, a ganglion cyst will need to be removed surgically.

CALL YOUR DOCTOR WHEN:

• you have pain in your wrist following a strenuous activity like tennis that is not relieved after two or three days of home treatment.

- you have had a fall or other sudden injury to your wrist that results in severe pain and/or deformity when compared to your normal wrist.
- you experience any weakness, numbness, or tingling in your hand or fingers as a result of a sprain or other wrist injury.
- you have what appears to be a ganglion on the back of your wrist that becomes persistent or bothersome.

HAND PAIN AND SYMPTOMS

DESCRIPTION

The human hand has been described by artists as the "perfect tool." Most hand pain and symptoms result from one of three problems: joint inflammation and swelling; nerve injuries causing weakness, numbness, and/or tingling of the fingers; and certain types of infections. Also, serious hand injuries such as cuts, dislocations, and fractures are usually painful and may result in permanent damage if not treated properly.

Joint inflammation and swelling usually come on gradually and can have dozens of causes. These include rheumatoid arthritis, osteoarthritis, gout, psoriasis, and infections. Each can affect the joints of the hand, and all require treatment.

Rheumatoid arthritis typically occurs between the ages of 25 and 50 and is two to three times more common in women than in men. It usually affects the joints of both hands as well as your other joints. Joint stiffness is often worse in the mornings or after prolonged inactivity. Although there is no cure, treatment can relieve pain and preserve function.

Another type of arthritis commonly causing symptoms of hand pain, swelling, and stiffness is called degenerative arthritis or osteoarthritis. This is the most common type of arthritis, especially in older folks, and, unlike rheumatoid arthritis, the pain is usually worse after exercise.

The nerves that control the delicate muscles that move your hand originate in the spinal cord in your neck (cervical spine). They branch beneath your armpit and course down your arm, through your wrist, and into your hand. Any injury to these nerves can cause symptoms of weakness, numbness, or tingling in your hands. Neck and shoulder injuries (*see* Shoulder Pain and Symptoms), dislocations, and elbow and wrist injuries also can cause these symptoms.

Most bacterial infections of the hand result from injuries that break the skin. Many infections also begin in the cuticle around the base of the fingernail (paronychia). Because the bones, muscles, and nerves in your hand are so delicate and so close together, infections spread quickly and may permanently damage these tissues.

Finally, hand injuries are a major cause of symptoms of pain, numbness, and tingling. The sudden onset of these symptoms should always cause concern. The small bones and tendons in the hand are easily fractured or dislocated, and the ligaments are easily torn. Cuts and abrasions, if not cleaned and treated properly, easily become infected, leading to long-term problems.

WHEN TO BE CONCERNED

Any hand symptoms beyond pain from minor cuts or abrasions require medical evaluation. Joint swelling and inflammation or any weakness, numbness, or tingling needs prompt attention before any permanent damage results.

If an infection doesn't respond promptly to a thorough cleaning and careful home treatment, see your doctor.

After a hand injury, even without significant pain, always consider the likelihood of a small fracture or dislocation. Any serious abrasion or deep cut may require stitches, and delays in treating these injuries can lead to infection and poor wound healing with scar tissue formation and loss of function.

TREATMENT

There is no one sure test for any type of arthritis, but blood tests and X-rays can help to evaluate your symptoms of joint inflammation and swelling. Rest, physical therapy, and aspirin are the most common treatments. Because the symptoms of arthritis are chronic, several new drugs with fewer side effects may be substituted for aspirin in long-term therapy. In severe cases, your doctor may suggest surgery to repair or replace the deformed joints.

Most symptoms of weakness, numbness, and tingling caused by a nerve injury are treated by correcting the underlying problem. If these symptoms are due to nerve pressure from a fracture or dislocation, your doctor will treat this injury first.

Treat small cuts and scratches by thoroughly cleaning the area and applying a topical antibiotic to prevent infection and a sterile dressing. If your tetanus immunization is current (*see* Immunizations), complications will be unlikely. Deeper cuts may require your wound to be cleaned surgically and stitched (sutured) to speed healing. Oral antibiotics may be necessary to prevent infection.

If you do develop an infection, see your doctor for treatment.

CALL YOUR DOCTOR WHEN:

- you have swelling, inflammation, or pain in the joints of your fingers that lasts longer than one week.
- you have weakness, numbness, or tingling in your hand with or without pain or a hand injury.
- you have a red, swollen, tender area around your cuticle or elsewhere on your hand that looks infected.
- you have a recent deep cut or a cut or abrasion that is not healing with home treatment.

LOW BACK PAIN AND SYMPTOMS

DESCRIPTION

If you have low back pain, you are in good company. Approximately 80 percent of all Americans experience such pain at one time or another. For most people, it occurs suddenly in the low back or lumbar region, often after bending, lifting, or even sneezing. Weakness of the muscles supporting your spine and poor posture account for most low back pain. Anatomical defects such as a tumor, fracture, herniated disc, or arthritis are responsible for back pain less than 15 percent of the time.

Repeated, uncomplicated low back pain also often results from obesity, a sedentary lifestyle, and poor muscle tone. These factors may often predispose you to injuries while engaging in weekend sports or other strenuous physical activities. Many who suffer from frequent recurrences often reinjure themselves during routine activities because of poor back care. In most of these cases, people incorrectly use their back to do the work of lifting instead of properly using their arms and legs.

WHEN TO BE CONCERNED

Your spinal column consists of 33 vertebrae supported by several muscles and ligaments. The nerves, including the sciatic nerve, pass between these vertebrae as they go from the spinal cord into the buttocks, trunk, and upper and lower extremities. Sciatica (pain radiating into your buttock, thigh, and lower leg) may sometimes accompany lower back pain. This sciatic pain may be associated with a ruptured or herniated disc. Irritation from pressure on the sciatic nerve may also cause painful spasm of the back and leg muscles. If your lower back pain is extended to your buttock, thigh, and lower leg, seek medical attention.

Most low back pain is recurrent, very similar each time, and is localized in the low back, rarely involving the sciatic nerve. But, if there is a sudden change in the character or severity of the pain or an extension of the pain along the sciatic nerve, see your doctor. Rarely, such symptoms may include weakness, numbness, or even paralysis of a lower extremity. If this occurs, you should seek *immediate* medical attention. You should also seek *immediate* medical evaluation if your low back pain occurs suddenly as a result of a fall or other trauma.

TREATMENT

Your treatment of uncomplicated low back pain may involve a regimen of bed rest for at least two or three days, aspirin or a similar painkiller taken every six hours, and hot baths twice daily. If your pain does not subside within a few days, or you develop additional symptoms, you should visit your doctor. After careful medical evaluation, your physician may prescribe a short course of muscle relaxants. If diagnostic tests show the cause of severe and continuous low back pain is due to tumor, nerve damage, or arthritis and inflammation of the vertebrae, you may require more intensive treatment, including a combination of surgery, drugs, and physical therapy.

In routine cases, after your acute pain subsides, you should begin back and abdominal strengthening exercises (*see* illustration of

EXERCISES FOR A BAD BACK

Before you begin any exercise program, consult with your doctor. Begin slowly, and increase the number of repetitions gradually. If any exercise causes or increases pain, discontinue it temporarily.

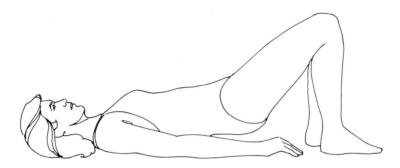

Pelvic Tilt

Lie flat on your back with knees bent. Pull in your stomach so that the small of your back is flat on the floor. Then, tighten your buttocks, and raise your hips. Hold for a count of 10. Repeat up to 20 times.

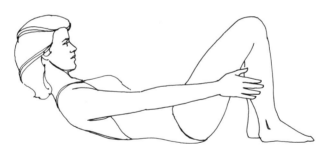

Bent-Leg Sit-Ups

Lie flat on your back. With the arms extended and legs bent, raise the trunk about 30 degrees off the floor. Relax. Repeat up to 20 times.

Knee-to-Forehead

Lie flat on your back with knees bent. Hold one knee with both hands and slowly bring it to the chest. At the same time, raise your shoulders off the floor and touch your forehead to the knee. Return slowly to the starting position. Repeat, alternating legs, up to 10 times.

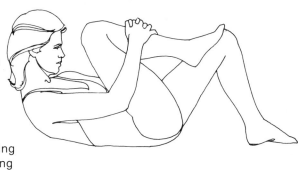

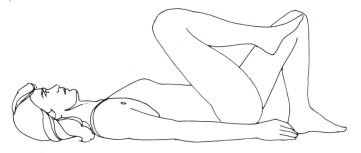

Lower Back Stretch

Lie flat on your back with knees bent, and slowly bring one knee as close to your chest as possible. Return it slowly to the starting position. Relax. Repeat up to 10 times for each leg.

Leg Raises

Lie flat on your back with knees bent. Bring one knee to the chest. Extend your leg upward, then bend your knee and return to the starting position. Relax. Repeat, alternating legs, up to 10 times.

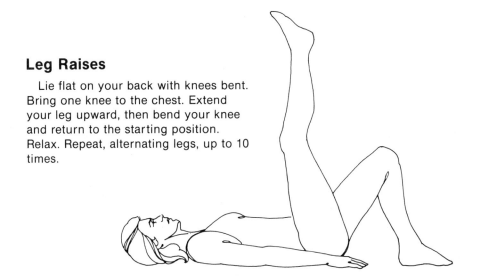

exercises for a bad back) as soon as possible. Both weight and stress reduction programs may also be helpful to you. Your posture should be checked carefully. When you lift objects, bend only at the knees, keeping your back upright and your stomach muscles tightened. You should avoid sports or other activities that require sudden body movements.

CALL YOUR DOCTOR WHEN:

- your pain is unrelieved after a few days of bed rest.
- your pain radiates into the buttock, thigh, or lower leg.
- your pain is the result of acute trauma.
- you experience numbness, weakness, or paralysis in your foot or leg (call immediately).

HIP PAIN AND SYMPTOMS

DESCRIPTION

Even though your thigh bone (femur) is the largest and strongest bone in your body, it may be subject to pain and stiffness as a result of arthritis, dislocation, fracture, or other injury.

Arthritis most commonly causes symptoms of hip pain, especially when there has been no injury. As you get older, routine wear and tear may cause the cartilage on the surfaces of your joints to become roughened. This degenerative arthritis (osteoarthritis) is common in older people and often affects the hip joints. The symptoms are a gradual stiffening that becomes painful when you stand or walk for any length of time. The pain usually will worsen after prolonged activity and improve somewhat with rest.

A hip fracture is another common cause of pain and other symptoms. This usually results from a fall. Hip fractures are especially serious in the elderly (see Special Health Concerns of Senior Citizens, Part I). Hip fractures often lead to serious complications such as strokes and pneumonia as well as poor and slow healing.

A rare cause of hip pain and stiffness is a dislocation. (The thighbone fits into a socket in your pelvis, forming the hip joint.)

Surprisingly, hip dislocation is usually caused by a fall on your foot or your knee. This serious injury is unusual because it takes great force to damage the strong ligaments that hold the end of your thighbone in its socket.

WHEN TO BE CONCERNED

Hip soreness from a new activity like skiing will usually go away by itself. But, if you gradually develop hip pain without an injury, and the pain continues for longer than a week or two, you should see your doctor.

Any fall by an elderly person that results in hip pain requires medical evaluation to rule out a fracture. If an injured person lying on his back is unable to lift his leg, suspect a hip fracture. Often the foot and leg on the injured side will be turned outward. A bruise over the hip, following a fall, is one clue to a likely fracture and should not be ignored. If a fracture is mistaken for a bruise, and the victim continues to hobble about in this condition, the bone will heal poorly and fail to provide adequate support. This often leads to another fall.

TREATMENT

If your hip pain comes on gradually, your doctor will carefully evaluate your symptoms and probably suggest X-rays to be certain that they are due to arthritis. If this is the cause, your most important treatment will be plenty of rest. Try to avoid strenuous or weight-bearing activities such as prolonged standing, climbing, or walking up and down a lot of steps. If you're overweight, lose weight to decrease the stress on your joints. Physical therapy may relieve some of your symptoms.

Your medical treatment will be similar to that described for arthritis (see Hand Pain and Symptoms). If you are otherwise active, and your arthritis is severe or painful and fails to respond to conservative treatment, your doctor may suggest a surgical hip replacement.

Although there is no cure for arthritis of the hip, adequate treatment may relieve your symptoms and enable you to enjoy a full and active life. If your arthritis shows only on an X-ray, but you feel fine, don't worry. We are all bound to suffer some wear and tear as we get older.

If you suspect a hip dislocation, never attempt to replace the thighbone in its socket. Get medical attention *immediately*. If ambulance care is not available, carefully place the victim on a firm board with a pillow under the knees and take him to an emergency room. Firmly support the leg and thigh during transport. Careful X-ray studies will be necessary, and anesthesia is almost always used in correcting the dislocation.

In treating a suspected hip fracture, turn the victim onto his back and gently place him on a long board. Carefully secure his body firmly to the board to steady the hip, pelvis, and spine. Transport him to an emergency room immediately. If a large board is not available, the victim's legs should be padded and bandaged tightly together. Move the injured leg as little as possible to avoid any further damage to nerves or blood vessels near the fracture. Your physician will generally want to order X-rays whenever a hip fracture is suspected since some fractures are difficult to detect.

CALL YOUR DOCTOR WHEN:

- you experience the gradual onset of hip pain or stiffness that persists for longer than a week or two.
- you have hip pain after a fall on your foot or knee.
- you have hip pain, a limp, or a bruise over your hip after a fall.
- you suspect a dislocation (*call immediately*).

LEG PAIN AND SYMPTOMS

DESCRIPTION

Most leg pain and other leg symptoms are due to cramps that originate in the muscles of your thigh and calf. Usually, there is no serious underlying cause. Occasionally, other more serious conditions (such as varicose veins or phlebitis) can cause similar symptoms of cramping or aching in your thigh and especially in your calf.

Muscle cramps are sudden, painful spasms that most often result from overexertion. A loss of body salts and/or a pulling or stretching of your leg muscles during exertion may be the reason for your cramps. Any strain on your leg muscles, such as wearing high-heeled shoes all day, can produce spasms. Chronic anxiety and stress may tighten your muscles and result in similar symptoms. Still another common cause is sciatica resulting from a low back injury (see Back Pain and Symptoms). Leg cramps may also accompany infections that cause high fever, chills, and sweating.

Varicose veins can give you both a cosmetic and an actual pain in your legs. The veins near the surface are usually involved and may become enlarged, bluish, twisted, and lumpy. These veins rarely cause severe symptoms, but in some cases you may experience increased soreness and fatigue. This condition is more common in women than in men and often occurs in families. It may be aggravated by pregnancy or obesity.

The most serious cause of thigh and calf pain is the formation of blood clots in the veins of the leg. While these may appear in the surface veins, they are much more serious when they occur in the deep veins. Small clots (emboli) sometimes break loose and travel through the bloodstream to the lung or brain, where they can cause a fatal blockage. If you have recently had pelvic or abdominal surgery, or you have injured or broken a lower limb, you are at high risk. Also, if you are taking birth control pills or have been bedridden for a prolonged period of time, you are prone to develop a blood clot.

WHEN TO BE CONCERNED

Almost everyone gets an occasional leg cramp. If your cramps are unrelated to a particular activity, appear repeatedly in the same spot, or follow a recent injury, you should see your doctor. If you have varicose veins, be concerned when a vein ruptures and bleeds after an injury or when an ulceration develops. Severe varicose veins should be checked by your doctor.

Most important, if you are at risk for blood clots, and you gradually develop severe pain, swelling, redness, or heaviness in your leg, get *immediate* medical attention. Be especially concerned if these symptoms are associated with any shortness of breath, chest pain, fever, or coughing blood. If leg swelling and pain develop after an injury or after being in bed for several days, you should also suspect a blood clot.

TREATMENT

Most ordinary leg cramps can be treated at home. Moist heat packs, massages, and rest are the mainstays. Physical therapy and exercise also may be helpful. If your pain persists or is severe, see your doctor. He'll check you thoroughly and possibly order some blood tests. He may prescribe medication for pain and muscle relaxants to relieve the spasm.

For most varicose veins that are mild to moderately severe, avoid prolonged standing and wear support hose. Also avoid tight clothing such as garters and girdles. Varicose veins that bleed or ulcerate require prompt medical attention. If your condition gets worse or complications develop, your doctor may recommend surgery or local injections to remove the affected veins.

You can prevent blood clots in your legs by reducing certain risk factors. If you have poor circulation, are pregnant, or have just had major surgery, take particular care to exercise your legs and keep them elevated. If you are bedridden for more than two or three days, use special support stockings to improve the circulation in your legs.

If you suspect a blood clot, there is no home treatment. Get *immediate* medical attention. The treatment for an early or mild blood clot will include bed rest with your feet elevated and aspirin or another anti-inflammatory medication. More serious cases may require hospitalization and drugs to thin your blood.

CALL YOUR DOCTOR WHEN:

- you have cramps in the same location that persist for several days without any apparent cause.
- you have varicose veins that are extremely painful or that bleed or ulcerate.
- you have any swelling, redness, or tenderness in your thigh or calf, especially if you are at risk of developing blood clots (*call immediately*).

KNEE PAIN AND SYMPTOMS

DESCRIPTION

Your knee is the largest and one of the most complex joints in your body, so it is very easily damaged. Most knee pain is the result of a sudden injury. It can also be due to arthritis or other conditions affecting all the bones and joints.

As in all your joints, the surfaces of the knee bones are lined with cartilage. This cartilage normally enables the bones to move smoothly against each other. There is one small cartilage on each side of your knee that supports this movement. A "locked knee" occurs when one or both of these cartilages is torn and gets caught in the joint. Your knee may lock or suddenly give way following an injury. Sometimes this occurs repeatedly in individuals who have these cartilages displaced. This condition is commonly called a "trick knee."

In addition to the cartilages that enable the bones in your knee joint to move smoothly over one another, your knee joint is also supported by several strong ligaments. As your knee normally flexes and extends, these strong ligaments prevent sideways motion and keep it stable as it supports your weight.

Though your knee joint is ordinarily extremely strong, it may be injured when a great strain is put on it. Any strain on your leg, from your ankle to your hip, may injure these ligaments. There are also ligaments above and below your kneecap (patella) that support it. Your kneecap protects the front of the knee joint.

WHEN TO BE CONCERNED

When your knee functions normally but suddenly gives out, suspect a possible torn cartilage. This is especially true if you have just suffered a twisting injury. You may hear a clicking sound when you try to move your knee. This is a clue that one or both of the cartilages is moving in and out of place. If your knee locks, and you feel a loose piece of cartilage in the joint, see your doctor promptly.

Any injury to your knee that results in severe pain, locking of the joint, or instability requires prompt medical attention. Since the ligaments and cartilages are often both damaged by a knee injury, any or all of these symptoms may be present. If you are totally unable to support your weight, suspect a torn ligament.

If you gradually develop any redness, swelling, or pain in your knee, even without a definite injury, you should also check with your doctor.

TREATMENT

If your knee is locking from a displaced cartilage, your doctor may try to manipulate it back into position. He may suggest splinting your knee to relieve the stress on the injured joint. If there is a lot of swelling, he may try to remove some of the fluid from the joint.

Your doctor may also request a special X-ray (arthrogram) of the knee joint to determine the extent of the damage to your cartilage. If the cartilage has actually been torn, the fragments of cartilage may be removed surgically and the joint repaired. This procedure has become fairly routine and generally will prevent a trick knee from developing.

Like the treatment of a locked knee due to a torn cartilage, torn ligaments often require surgical repair. If you suspect a serious knee injury, splint your knee immediately and get prompt medical attention. Avoid bearing weight on the injured knee. When you see your doctor, be sure to tell him how your injury occurred. Many times, this will clearly help him determine which ligaments or cartilages have been injured.

Torn ligaments causing severe pain may be treated with the injection of local anesthetic and with oral painkillers. Again, if there is significant swelling, your doctor may try to remove some of the fluid. If the ligament is only strained, your knee should be splinted for at least two weeks. If it is actually ruptured, the doctor may recommend a plaster cast for a much longer time to be certain that the ligament heals properly. Many orthopedic surgeons prefer immediate surgical treatment of torn ligaments.

CALL YOUR DOCTOR WHEN:

- your knee suddenly locks after an injury, and you are unable to flex or extend it.
- you feel a piece of cartilage moving in your knee.
- you have pain or swelling around your knee after an injury.
- you are unable to support your weight after a knee injury.
- you have any redness, pain, or swelling of your knee joint, even in the absence of injury.

ANKLE PAIN AND SYMPTOMS

DESCRIPTION

Like any other joint in your body, your ankle may gradually become painful from any of the causes of arthritis mentioned earlier (*see* Generalized Bone and Joint Swelling and Pain). Most sudden, severe ankle pain results from an acute injury such as a strain or sprain. A strain is a mild stress on a muscle or tendon; a sprain is the stretching or actual tearing of a ligament.

Some orthopedists consider a severe ankle sprain to be worse than an outright fracture. Severely torn ligaments heal slowly and often poorly, which may lead to repeated ankle sprains.

It is extremely rare for your ankle to become dislocated without an accompanying fracture. Most fractures are actually caused indirectly by a force applied to your foot and transmitted to your ankle. Usually, this force turns your foot either inward or outward, each causing a different type of fracture. Your ankle joint is very complicated and involves the union of several bones and ligaments. Because of this, in severe ankle injuries, more than one bone is often fractured.

WHEN TO BE CONCERNED

You can't always judge the severity of an injury by your pain. Sometimes a mild ankle sprain, with a partially torn ligament, is more painful than a completely torn ligament. See your doctor if you have any significant pain or swelling or can't support your weight comfortably after an ankle injury. Splint or tape the ankle with an elastic bandage and avoid bearing weight on it. You may apply cold packs to relieve the swelling.

Basically, any sudden twisting injury causing severe pain and swelling should suggest a fracture until proven otherwise. Compare your injured ankle to your normal ankle. Any deformity or displacement of the bone is a clue to a likely ankle fracture and requires prompt medical evaluation.

TREATMENT

Your doctor will check your ankle and lower leg and suggest X-rays to determine the extent of injury to the bones and ligaments. Mild ankle strains and sprains without a torn ligament do not require a cast. More severe sprains often require a cast to steady the ankle joint while the ligaments heal. A completely torn ligament usually requires a walking cast for at least six weeks to promote healing and to prevent a recurrence. Avoid putting any stress on your ankle for several weeks afterward.

Occasionally, when X-rays show that a ligament is completely torn, your doctor may advise surgery to repair the tear. This is especially true if you are young and extremely active in sports. Follow your doctor's advice carefully to prevent long-term weakness and repeated ankle sprains. It may take as long as three to four months until your ankle has completely returned to normal.

If you suspect an ankle fracture, seek medical attention as soon as possible. Avoid bearing weight on it, apply cold packs, and splint and elevate the ankle during transport to an emergency room. Most experts recommend that you splint the injured ankle with the shoe on and wrap the lower third of your leg with an elastic bandage.

Ankle fractures almost always require some type of cast, with the period of time depending on the extent of your injury. Severe fractures that impair the blood supply to your foot or where the bone fragments are sufficiently dislocated to prevent normal healing may require surgery. After your cast is on for about 24 hours, you'll need to return to the doctor to be sure that there is good circulation to your foot and toes.

CALL YOUR DOCTOR WHEN:

- you have severe ankle swelling and pain following a sudden injury.
- you are unable to walk comfortably or have any numbness or tingling in your foot several hours after an injury.
- you gradually develop pain, redness, or swelling in your ankle that persists for more than two days, even without an injury.

FOOT PAIN AND SYMPTOMS

DESCRIPTION

Most people overlook the importance of their feet. Anything that causes foot problems will likely put a crimp in your lifestyle. Corns, calluses, bunions, diseases of the joints of the feet (such as gout), fungal infections such as athlete's foot (tinea pedis), and ingrown toenails are all capable of producing enough pain to keep you from walking. Your feet, and especially your toes, may also be accidently injured. A "stubbed toe" is usually nothing to worry about, but untreated fracture of the small bones of the foot and toes can lead to permanent disability.

If you have bunions, you probably got them because you wear shoes that are too tight. Over time, pressure from tight shoes produces redness and irritation (inflammation) near the joint of the big toe. Continued friction over the joint causes the bone to harden and become inflexible. A large, bony growth develops, usually on the inner side of the big toe. Women get bunions more often than men and generally develop them in both feet. Once you have bunions, you may have difficulty finding shoes that fit. Your worst symptom, however, will be pain.

Areas of hard, thickened skin are called either corns or calluses. They develop on an area where there is repeated or prolonged pressure or friction. Corns tend to be pea-sized or slightly larger. They are usually tender and typically occur on your feet either between the toes (soft corns) or over the bony areas (hard corns).

Calluses are less tender and usually have less definite margins than corns. The palms of your hands and the soles of your feet are the most common sites, but they can develop anyplace where there is pressure. For example, guitarists have calluses on their fingers, and violinists get them under their chins. Because both corns and calluses occur on the soles of your feet, you may confuse them with plantar warts (see Skin Discolorations).

Gout typically occurs as a sudden attack causing pain, redness, and swelling of the joint of the big toe. The wrist, ankle, knee, and even your thumb may be involved. Later attacks may be less intense but often last longer. After time, the disease can cause crystals of uric acid to deposit in tissue around your joints, causing stiffness and deformity. Gout is inherited, with 90 percent of the sufferers male, usually over age 30.

Fungal infections can affect either the skin of your feet, causing athlete's foot, or the toenails. Both infections are actually a form of ringworm. Athlete's foot is a common problem that causes itching and burning between the toes and on the soles of your feet. After a long time, it is not unusual for your toenails to become infected as well. Athlete's foot is highly contagious and can be spread by direct contact or by using an infected person's towel or shoes.

Most people get ingrown toenails from either chronic irritation or manicuring too closely to the nail edge. Once the nail becomes ingrown, there is a danger of infection. The area around the toenail becomes red, swollen, and tender to touch.

WHEN TO BE CONCERNED

Any persistent pain following a foot injury should receive prompt medical attention.

If a bunion becomes so painful that you are unable to walk, see your doctor. If you suffer from diabetes or poor circulation, you should never remove corns or calluses on your own because of the increased risk of infection. Although most cases of athlete's foot tend to be mild and self-limited, a diabetic who develops a foot infection (fungal infection or ingrown toenail) should seek prompt medical attention. Rarely, a severely infected ingrown toenail will spread more deeply into the tissues of the toe, affecting the tendons and even the bone.

The most serious complication of gout is kidney failure. Chronic arthritis is another complication. Although no one really knows why, people with gout have an increased incidence of high blood pressure (hypertension), kidney disease, diabetes, high fats (triglycerides) in the blood, and hardening of the arteries (atherosclerosis).

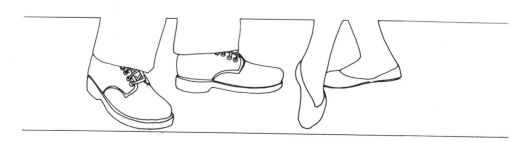

TREATMENT

Most foot injuries can be prevented by wearing the proper shoes for each activity. If your doctor determines that you have fractured your foot he will recommend a cast or special shoe to aid in healing. A broken toe is usually treated by taping it to the adjacent toe until it has healed.

You can prevent bunions, corns, and calluses on your feet by wearing shoes that fit properly. If you already have bunions, you can relieve the pain by enlarging or cutting your shoes. This will eliminate pressure on your bunions. Some specialized shoe stores sell "bunion last" shoes with a wide forefoot section. Or you may want to have shoes custom-made. Whenever possible, avoid wearing high-heeled, narrow-toed shoes. If your pain is not relieved by these techniques, consult your physician. You may be a candidate for surgery. However, before you decide on surgery, you should get a second opinion and make sure you understand the risks.

Once you have a corn or callus, try soaking the area in hot water. Or you may apply a softening agent such as salicylic acid. Purchase this at your pharmacy and carefully follow the enclosed directions (do not apply the agent to normal skin). A few days after applying this preparation, use an emery board to remove the thickened dead skin. If your callus or corn is on a weight-bearing area, ask your pharmacist for a metatarsal bar or foam pad to help relieve the pressure.

The aim of the treatment for gout is to minimize the formation of uric acid crystals; your doctor may prescribe any of several different drugs to do so once he has made the diagnosis. A high liquid intake will help to increase your daily urine output. Special diets haven't been shown to affect attacks.

Good foot hygiene is essential for the prevention of fungal

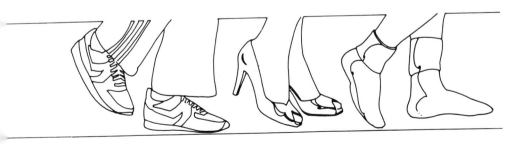

infections. Keep your feet clean and dry, especially in warm weather. In warm weather, wear light shoes such as sandals that allow air to circulate between your toes. Over-the-counter medications specifically labeled for athlete's foot may be helpful in mild cases, but they usually don't work on your toenails. Check with your doctor if you have a severe or chronic case of athlete's foot or the nails are involved. He may examine a skin scraping and prescribe an oral antifungal drug.

If you have an ingrown toenail that does not appear to be infected, try soaking your toe in hot water. However, if there is redness, swelling, and severe pain with or without pus, consult your physician. He may need to open the area near the toenail surgically to drain the infection. It is also likely that he will prescribe antibiotics.

CALL YOUR DOCTOR WHEN:

- you have any persistent pain following a foot injury.
- you have a bunion that is so painful that it interferes with your walking.
- you have a painful corn or callus, an ingrown toenail, or a fungal infection of your feet and you have diabetes or poor circulation.
- you have an infected ingrown toenail.
- you notice a sudden painful swelling and redness of any of your joints, especially the big toe.

Chapter 7

Symptoms and Diseases of the Brain and Nervous System

ANXIETY

DESCRIPTION

Anxiety is a common, temporary feeling of nervousness, worry, or fear that may be appropriate for a situation and may actually serve a useful purpose. Anxiety before a race, for example, may prepare you physically to compete by increasing your breathing and heart rate. Anxiety that occurs only in a specific situation—in elevators, for example—is called a phobia.

Some people, anxious for no reason at all, are said to have "free-floating anxiety." When this becomes chronic, it may interfere with work and social life and cause a variety of symptoms, including fatigue, muscle tension (especially headaches), and decreased appetite. These people are often convinced that they have a serious illness and that they should seek a medical evaluation of their symptoms. Occasionally, symptoms of anxiety also occur with illnesses such as an overactive thyroid gland or heart disease.

WHEN TO BE CONCERNED

If you are overanxious, you may experience difficulty swallowing, profound sweating, diarrhea, vague chest pain, irregular heartbeat (palpitations), muscle twitching, or insomnia. You may breathe fast (hyperventilate) and become light-headed, dizzy, and even faint. Report any of these symptoms to your doctor.

TREATMENT

Treatment of anxiety may simply involve avoiding these situations or learning to overcome a phobia. Relaxation or behavior modification techniques may work. Exercise or a warm bath may relax tense muscles. Avoid caffeine, chocolate, cigarettes, and drugs, which may make you feel anxious. If you are hyperventilating, breathe into a paper bag until your breathing returns to normal. Severe anxiety may require therapy with a psychologist or psychiatrist and possibly prescribed medication.

CALL YOUR DOCTOR WHEN:

- your anxiety is chronic and interferes with your daily life.
- you experience sweating, difficulty swallowing, diarrhea, irregular heartbeat, chest pain, muscle twitching, insomnia, light-headedness, dizziness, or fainting.

PERSONALITY CHANGE

DESCRIPTION

Everybody gets the blues. Being sad or feeling depressed is a normal way for you to respond to certain disappointments or losses. For example, some people feel down around holidays (especially if they're away from home and family); others feel low on the anniversary of a loved one's death. Women may feel this way just before menstruation or just after childbirth.

Anytime you are sick, you may have associated feelings of depression. These reactions to specific stressful or unhappy life situations may occur at any age, from infancy through old age. They are usually temporary and not serious. However, if these feelings continue for several weeks or more and begin to interfere with your normal functioning, you may be suffering from a type of depression that requires professional help.

How do you know if you are suffering from this kind of depression? Typically, depression affects your sleep pattern, your appetite, your energy level, your mood, and your thoughts. But while one person may have trouble falling asleep or staying asleep (insomnia) with depression, another may feel like sleeping all the time; some people become hyperactive, while others can't seem to find the energy to do anything. Even moods may be different between two individuals who are both depressed. One may appear terribly sad, while the other may hide his feelings behind a smile (masked depression). Some people with depression have violent mood swings, alternating between being very elated and very down (manic depression). It is not unusual for people with depression to have trouble concentrating or making decisions.

Anorexia nervosa and bulimia are two serious eating disorders often associated with depression. In both conditions, the victims (usually young women) are preoccupied with food and losing weight. The difference is how they lose weight.

People with anorexia go on very strict diets, including fasting, despite normal appetites. They may also exercise compulsively. Even after reaching their ideal weight, they're not satisfied because they still see a fat person when they look in the mirror. So they keep dieting, often until they become severely malnourished. Without treatment, the disorder may be fatal.

Bulimics typically eat tremendous amounts of high-calorie foods (binging) and then try to get rid of the food through forced vomiting or laxative use (purging). This binging and purging can occur daily, weekly, or only occasionally. Excessive vomiting can cause serious gum disease and nutritional deficiencies.

WHEN TO BE CONCERNED

If you are severely depressed, you may have thoughts of hopelessness and failure. You may withdraw from relationships with your family or friends, lose interest in the pleasures of daily living, and even think about suicide. If you experience any of these symptoms, see your doctor *immediately*.

Children tend to deal with depression by complaining of head-

COMMON SIGNS AND SYMPTOMS OF DEPRESSION

- change in sleep pattern (insomnia or staying in bed)
- change in appetite (marked increase or decrease)
- hyperactivity or underactivity
- loss of usual interests (including decreased interest in sex)

- withdrawal from relationships
- trouble concentrating or making decisions
- feelings of hopelessness and failure
- mood swings (manic/depressive)
- thoughts of suicide

aches or stomach pain with no apparent physical cause, by refusing to see friends, through self-destructive behavior such as tantrums or neglecting schoolwork.

If you have become so preoccupied with food, your eating habits, and/or your weight that you diet and exercise compulsively or binge and purge, you may have an eating disorder and should consult your doctor.

TREATMENT

The treatment of your depression depends on its cause and severity. If the cause is psychological, your doctor will probably recommend counseling along with antidepressant medication. If the cause is physical, your doctor will make a diagnosis and treat appropriately. Rarely, you may need to be hospitalized.

If you have an eating disorder, you are not alone. Many people have similar difficulties. Discuss this with your doctor. He may suggest group or individual therapy combined with weight control, using behavior modification methods. Extreme weight loss and malnutrition may require temporary hospitalization.

CALL YOUR DOCTOR WHEN:

- you have thoughts of suicide (*call immediately*).
- you experience signs and symptoms of depression (*see* Common Signs and Symptoms of Depression), especially for more than a few weeks.
- you suspect you have an eating disorder.

MEMORY LOSS, CONFUSION, AND DELIRIUM

DESCRIPTION

You've probably joked about getting old whenever you've forgotten something, but the truth is, not all of us lose our memory as we age. In fact, disorders of your mental state (confusion and delirium as well as memory loss) may be symptoms of serious brain disease. Causes also include alcohol and drug intoxication, drug withdrawal, infections, malnutrition, head injury, severe epilepsy, and cancer.

It's perfectly normal to forget things from time to time. However, loss of memory of recent rather than past events may not be.

Often, a serious memory problem will be accompanied by impairment of other intellectual functions as well. A person may appear confused and not know who or where he is. He may not know the year, the month, or the day of the week. He may cry or laugh without reason and may be very depressed or anxious. This usually occurs when the individual realizes that he has a problem and reacts with anger and denial.

Delirium is a temporary mental disturbance that begins suddenly with disorientation. People who are delirious seem restless and anxious. They tend to mistake the unfamiliar for the familiar. For example, they may mistake hospital for home, nurses for family members. Delirium is a symptom of many disorders, including alcoholic intoxication (DTs), infections, brain tumor, exhaustion, high fever, and malnutrition. The condition is thought to result from a chemical imbalance in the brain.

WHEN TO BE CONCERNED

Normal forgetfulness is nothing to worry about. However, when you or someone in your family develops a memory loss only for recent events, especially if associated with other symptoms such as confusion and disorientation, you should consult your physician. Whenever these symptoms come on suddenly, see your doctor *immediately.*

TREATMENT

To treat memory loss, confusion, or delirium, the underlying cause must be diagnosed and treated. Your doctor will do a complete physical examination and may perform certain tests, including an electroencephalogram (EEG) and/or a CAT scan. If the cause is reversible, prompt diagnosis and treatment will improve recovery of mental function. Anyone who is delirious should be protected from injury until you get him or her to a doctor. Remember to bring any medications the individual may be taking.

CALL YOUR DOCTOR WHEN:

• you or someone in your family suffers from loss of memory of recent events, especially if associated with confusion and disorientation.
• these symptoms come on suddenly (*call immediately*).

LOSS OF CONSCIOUSNESS

DESCRIPTION

If you experience a sudden loss of consciousness, it may be brief, as in a faint, or prolonged, as in a coma. Your brain requires a constant, uninterrupted supply of oxygen. Whenever there is a decrease in the amount of blood that carries oxygen to your brain, you will suddenly lose consciousness. This can happen when your heart rate suddenly slows and causes a drop in your blood pressure. This reflex may be triggered by fear, anxiety, pain, extreme hunger, or fatigue. Even being in a hot, crowded room too long may cause you to faint.

Simple fainting (vasovagal syncope) is your body's way of telling you to lie down in order to increase the supply of oxygen-filled blood to your brain. Typically, you will be standing or sitting when the faint occurs. A sudden loss of consciousness may be preceded by muscle weakness, increasing heart rate, a cold sweat, and pallor (*see* Skin Discolorations). Minutes later, you may feel light-headed and notice blurred vision before actually fainting. In these cases of a simple faint, merely lying down will normally quickly restore consciousness. If you don't lie down immediately, you may experience a brief but mild convulsion (*see* Convulsions).

Some people are very sensitive to changes in their blood pressure and will faint just from rising too quickly from a sitting or lying position. This is especially true when someone who has been bedridden for several days tries to get up for the first time.

Coma is complete and prolonged unconsciousness from which someone can't be aroused. Coma has many causes, including severe head or brain injury, stroke, severe diabetes, tumors, shock, and drug overdose. *It is always a medical emergency.*

WHEN TO BE CONCERNED

An isolated simple faint, especially when there is an obvious cause, is usually nothing to worry about. If you become faint from being in a hot, crowded room for too long, from extreme fright, or from being upset about something, chances are this is a simple faint. Occasionally, however, more serious problems may cause you to faint. Certain types of heart disease, severe anemia, diabetes, hypoglycemia, drug overdoses, and epilepsy can all cause sudden loss of consciousness. Whenever you experience a convulsion or a head injury associated with fainting or the faint can't be explained on the basis of a particular situation, promptly consult your physician. Recurring fainting always requires prompt medical evaluation.

Coma is always a medical emergency and may occur in many diseases just before death. Anytime you are unable to arouse someone, call an ambulance *immediately.*

TREATMENT

When you witness someone faint, place the person on his or her back with the head lower than the rest of the body. Loosen any tight clothing and be sure the victim gets plenty of fresh air. You may try using smelling salts, but some doctors feel that this may irritate the nasal passages and occasionally cause vomiting.

If you feel as though you might faint, lie down the moment you notice any early warning signs (muscle weakness, increased heart rate, cold sweat, pallor, light-headedness, blurred vision). If you can't lie down, sit with your head between your knees and breathe deeply.

To evaluate your fainting, your doctor will need a thorough history to determine what brought on this symptom. Try to recall all of your other symptoms. Bring any medication you are taking with you, since your symptoms may be caused by a drug reaction, which is especially common with certain high blood pressure pills. After a careful physical examination, your doctor may order X-rays and other special tests, including an electrocardiogram (EKG). Once he has determined the cause of your symptoms, he will be able to recommend appropriate treatment.

Since coma is a medical emergency, it is always handled in the hospital and involves diagnosis and treatment of the underlying cause.

CALL YOUR DOCTOR WHEN:

- you experience a fainting episode that can't be explained on the basis of a particular situation or emotion.
- your fainting is associated with a head injury or convulsion.
- you have a serious disease (such as diabetes or heart disease) and faint.
- you have recurrent fainting episodes.
- you are unable to arouse someone who is unconscious (*call immediately*).

CONVULSIONS

DESCRIPTION

If you've ever seen someone having a convulsion (also known as a seizure or fit), you know it can be pretty frightening. Convulsions are involuntary muscle contractions that cause contortions of the body and limbs. There are many different kinds of convulsions, from a slight fluttering of the eyes and blank staring (petit mal), to generalized convulsions (grand mal), associated with tongue biting, abnormal breathing, and possibly loss of bowel or bladder control.

There are also many different causes of convulsions. Just as fever is a symptom of certain diseases, convulsions are a clue to an underlying disease or abnormality. Not all convulsions are caused by epilepsy; they may be caused by high fever, alcohol withdrawal, drug overdose, low blood sugar (hypoglycemia), infections such as meningitis, head injuries, strokes, brain tumors, and other conditions.

Epilepsy is a brain disorder that affects about 2 percent of the population. It usually begins between ages 2 and 14. After the first convulsion, others may occur from time to time. These may be the result of sudden temporary changes in the electrical activity of the brain, but in most cases the cause of these changes is unknown. One thing is certain: whatever the cause, people with epilepsy are usually normal between attacks, and today most attacks can be prevented with medication.

In the very young, convulsions may be brought on by a high fever (febrile convulsions). A sudden rise in temperature, usually to 104 degrees Fahrenheit or higher, may trigger a convulsion in a normal child. However, seizures may run in the family. About a third of children who have this type of febrile convulsion will have more seizures later in life even without a fever.

Certain infections that affect the brain and are associated with high fever may be the cause of convulsions. Fever and neck stiffness suggest possible meningitis and should be treated *immediately* by a physician.

Finally, anytime someone has been a heavy alcohol drinker and then suddenly stops drinking (alcohol withdrawal), there may be symptoms that include generalized convulsions ("rum fits"). These usually occur about 12-48 hours after the drinking stopped.

WHEN TO BE CONCERNED

Whenever you or someone in your family experiences a convulsion for the first time, you should consult a physician. Sometimes, people with a known seizure disorder that was controlled with medicine begin having seizures again. This is often due to a problem with the dosage of their medication. Check with your doctor.

Convulsions are of particular concern when they are prolonged since they may result in brain damage. Anytime someone develops convulsions that don't stop after several minutes or seems to be having one convulsion after the other (status epilepticus), you should call an ambulance immediately. *This is a medical emergency.*

TREATMENT

The treatment of convulsions will depend on their cause. The diagnosis requires a thorough history, a careful physical examination, and selected laboratory tests. Often the person who has had the seizure will experience forgetfulness (amnesia) after an attack, so whenever possible, bring an eyewitness with you to the doctor.

How the convulsion began, what it looked like, how long it lasted, whether there was tongue biting or loss of bowel or bladder control, and whether there was sleepiness afterward are all questions your doctor will ask. Also try to recall whether you experienced any sensation (aura) just before the seizure, such as seeing, hearing, or smelling something strange or unpleasant. If the convulsion seemed to occur just after eating a certain food, drinking alcohol, taking any medication, seeing lights, hearing sounds, or stress, this may be a clue. Also tell your doctor if you have a family history of convulsions.

Depending on your history and examination, your doctor may order an X-ray of your skull, an electroencephalogram (EEG), a lumbar puncture (LP), and/or a CAT scan.

If your diagnosis is epilepsy, you will be treated with certain medications. Drugs can control seizures in most cases. Follow your doctor's instructions carefully. He will probably need to check your blood from time to time to see that your dosage is correct. Learn about side effects and immediately report any you experience.

Even if you do have epilepsy, there is no reason why you can't live a normal life. Eat properly, get plenty of rest, and try to eliminate as much stress from your life as possible. Of course, be sure to check with your doctor first, but if you are well controlled, you should be able to do anything anyone else can do—swim, dance, even ride horseback. Most state licensing agencies permit driving after the convulsions have stopped for one year.

If someone in your family has epilepsy, treat the person the way you'd treat anyone that you loved. Be sympathetic, but not too overprotective. People with epilepsy are rarely retarded. In fact, they may have above-average intelligence, and they are usually perfectly able to live normal lives.

If your child has a convulsion associated with high fever, call your doctor *immediately*. Once the episode is treated, your doctor may decide to keep your child on medication for a few years.

Seizures due to infections, alcohol withdrawal, drug overdose, head injury, or stroke require emergency treatment. If you happen to observe someone having a convulsion, place something firm but soft (like a folded handkerchief) between the person's teeth. Loosen any clothing around the neck. If there has been head and especially neck injury, don't move the person's neck. Otherwise, put the person in a position to prevent him from inhaling his own vomit. Make sure the victim is breathing and has a heartbeat. If not, immediately start cardiopulmonary resuscitation (CPR) and have someone call for an ambulance.

CALL YOUR DOCTOR WHEN:

- you or someone in your family experiences a convulsion for the first time.
- you have a diagnosed seizure disorder and your seizures are not controlled by the medicine you are taking.
- someone has a prolonged convulsion or one convulsion after the other *(call immediately—this is a medical emergency)*.

DIZZINESS

DESCRIPTION

You've probably heard someone call another person "dizzy," meaning that the person is a little foolish or even stupid. That's because the word dizzy comes from an old English word, *dysig*, which means just that. However, when you say that *you* feel dizzy, you usually are trying to say that you feel light-headed or giddy. In this strict sense, dizziness is very different from vertigo, in which you experience the illusion of movement (either you feel yourself moving or you think things around you are moving) (*see* Dizziness, Vertigo, or Loss of Consciousness).

The most common cause of dizziness is physical or emotional strain. For example, after playing a strenuous game of tennis in the hot sun, you might experience some light-headedness, especially if you've been sweating a lot and haven't been watching your fluid or salt intake. Likewise, as part of an acute anxiety reaction, you may suddenly feel light-headed and actually faint (*see* Loss of Consciousness).

Although dizziness is often nothing to worry about, it may also result from low blood sugar (hypoglycemia), drug reactions, alcohol intoxication, or head injury.

WHEN TO BE CONCERNED

If you're feeling a little light-headed when you are too warm, overtired, tense, or nervous, and the episode lasts for just a few moments, chances are there is nothing to worry about. However, whenever you experience prolonged dizziness or recurrent dizzy spells, you should consult your physician. Occasionally, dizziness may be caused by medication you are taking (especially drugs for high blood pressure), so check with your doctor.

You've probably heard about hypoglycemia and know it can cause dizziness, but you may not realize that dizziness alone is generally not caused by low blood sugar. If you have other symptoms, such as sudden blurred or double vision, headache, irritability, sweating, and palpitations, suspect hypoglycemia and call your doctor *immediately*. This reaction may occur if you are a diabetic and take too much insulin, wait too long to eat, exercise too much, or just don't eat enough food. Healthy people who drink alcohol on an empty stomach or who drink alcohol mixed with sugar-containing mixers may also develop symptoms of hypoglycemia.

Anytime you experience dizziness associated with a head injury with or without loss of consciousness, call your doctor.

TREATMENT

The treatment of dizziness depends on the cause of your symptoms. If you know your dizziness is related to certain stressful emotional situations, try to avoid them or consider counseling to overcome your anxiety. If your dizziness is associated with being overtired, often a brief period of rest will solve your problem.

Anytime you experience dizziness with other symptoms suggesting hypoglycemia, you can try eating sugar or sugar-containing food such as honey, candy, or fruit. However, even if you feel better, you should see your doctor for a complete evaluation. Don't forget to take along any medications you are taking and be prepared to explain exactly what seems to bring on your symptoms. That's the best way for your doctor to make an accurate diagnosis.

CALL YOUR DOCTOR WHEN:

- your dizziness doesn't go away within a short time.
- you experience recurrent episodes of dizziness.
- your dizziness is associated with a head injury (*call immediately*).
- your dizziness is associated with symptoms suggesting hypoglycemia.

LOCALIZED WEAKNESS

DESCRIPTION

Many people confuse symptoms of weakness, fatigue, and exhaustion (*see* Weakness, Fatigue, and Exhaustion). Localized weakness is really an actual loss of muscle strength in one muscle or muscle group.

Since weakness is a relative symptom, always describe it to your doctor carefully in terms of your normal activities. The muscles involved will give your doctor a clue to the underlying cause. For example, if one side of your face is weak (*see* Paralysis), your doctor will know that a particular nerve and muscle group is involved. Weakness of the same muscles on both sides of your body is likely emotional or caused by a generalized illness. Weakness clearly localized in one arm or one leg is more likely caused by a nerve or muscle injury.

Your other symptoms may provide additional clues. Numbness and tingling in any weakened limb are likely due to a nerve injury. Fever or weight loss, on the other hand, suggest a general underlying illness as the cause of your weakness. Pain in the weakened muscle group is a clue that the muscles themselves may be involved.

WHEN TO BE CONCERNED

Weakness in a particular muscle group that limits your regular activity is a significant symptom. Is there a change in the size of your muscles? Compare the weakened muscle with the opposite normal muscle. Any change in size or muscle mass is significant. Any associated weight loss, fever, or numbness and tingling in the weakened muscle is a cause for concern.

TREATMENT

There is basically no home treatment for significant weakness in a particular muscle group. Don't simply try exercises to increase strength. See your doctor promptly and give him a very careful medical history. He'll watch you perform various tasks with the weakened muscles, check your reflexes, and measure your strength. Certain blood tests, nerve conduction studies, and possibly a muscle biopsy may be necessary to find the cause.

CALL YOUR DOCTOR WHEN:

• you experience any significant localized weakness in any part of your body.

PARALYSIS

DESCRIPTION

You probably think of the inability to move the arms or legs when you hear the word paralysis, but that's not entirely accurate. The word paralysis refers to loss of movement of *any* muscle of your body. You can experience paralysis of just the muscles of one side of your face, as in a condition called Bell's palsy, or one whole side of your body, as in the case of some strokes. Parkinson's disease (paralysis agitans) is not a true form of paralysis. With this disorder, people move their muscles so slowly that they may appear to be paralyzed.

Bell's palsy typically comes on suddenly and for no apparent reason. It's possible that sleeping with your windows open and getting a chill could produce this disorder, but that's really only a theory. Whatever the reason, the nerve that controls the muscles of half the face is affected, resulting in paralysis. The involved side will look flat, and when you smile, only the unaffected side moves, so your expression may seem twisted. In severe cases, you may have trouble closing one eye. Often there is a decreased sensation on the affected side as well.

Strokes (cerebrovascular accidents) can occur whenever the blood supply to your brain is decreased. They are extremely rare in people under 40. Usually the cause is a clot or plug somewhere in the vessels of your neck or brain that blocks the flow of blood to your brain. This can also happen anytime a clot dislodges from your heart or the arteries leading to the head and is carried into the smaller arteries of the brain. Bleeding inside the brain itself can also result in damage to brain tissue. Typically, a stroke occurs suddenly. Depending on what area of the brain is affected, it may produce symptoms from slight slurring of speech to paralysis of one side of your body to coma.

Parkinson's disease generally affects middle-aged and elderly people. Rather than paralysis, the disease begins with a tremor, usually in one hand, followed by slowing of movement and finally rigidity of muscles.

WHEN TO BE CONCERNED

Anytime you experience paralysis of any muscle, consult your physician. Don't ignore symptoms that come and go since they may be a clue to something more serious. Although strokes are the third leading cause of death in the United States, attention to warning signs such as temporary loss of movement in the limbs of one side of your body, changes in speech or vision, or occasional fainting spells can lead to stroke prevention.

TREATMENT

Most cases of Bell's palsy are not severe and will resolve within a few weeks to a few months without specific treatment. If your eye is involved, your doctor may recommend methylcellulose eye drops and/or an eye patch to protect the cornea. Upward massage of the face for 5-10 minutes three to four times a day may help to maintain muscle tone.

You can prevent strokes if you control your blood pressure, stop smoking, and watch the fats in your diet (*see* Types of Fats, Part I). Studies have shown that women taking birth control pills have a higher risk of developing strokes, so if you are over 35, have migraine headaches, or have a family history of strokes, use another form of contraception.

If you have any of the warning signs of impending stroke, see your doctor *immediately*. He may recommend taking aspirin every day. Experts feel this may help to prevent clots from forming in your blood vessels. However, never take any drug, including aspirin, without checking with your doctor first. Once you actually have a stroke, your doctor will prescribe therapy based on your disability. Don't be discouraged. Recovery is often remarkably complete. If you have any paralysis of your muscles, your physician will probably recommend physical therapy. If your speech is affected, he will likely suggest speech therapy.

CALL YOUR DOCTOR WHEN:

- you experience paralysis of any muscle.
- you have temporary loss of movement in any muscle with or without other symptoms.

HEADACHE

DESCRIPTION

Headaches are probably the single most common symptom that brings people to their doctor. While a headache can be extremely painful, its severity is not related to its seriousness. For example, migraine headaches are extremely painful but usually not very serious. On the other hand, a brain tumor may sometimes cause only a mild headache.

Fortunately, most headaches are not serious and are relieved with home treatment. These are typically tension headaches caused by muscle spasm and related directly to stress. They usually occur during the day and cause a tightness or pressure sensation over your forehead, at your temples, or at the back of your neck.

Like tension headaches, migraine headaches tend to run in families. Migraines are thought to be caused by a disturbance in the blood vessels of the head and neck and are thus known as vascular headaches. Before a migraine headache, you may experience visual disturbances, depression, irritability or other characteristic symptoms. The headache itself is often described as a throbbing pain located on one side of the head. Unlike tension headaches, migraines usually are accompanied by nausea and vomiting. Without treatment, attacks may last for hours or days.

Besides tension and migraines, there are many other causes of headache symptoms, including fever; head injuries; dental disease; diseases of the eyes (such as eyestrain or glaucoma), ears (such as middle ear infections), or of the nasal sinuses (such as sinusitis); severe high blood pressure; allergies; and exposure to certain toxic substances (such as carbon monoxide or lead).

HEAD INJURY PRECAUTIONS

If you have suffered a hard blow or bump to your head, you should be aware of danger signs that indicate the need for prompt medical attention. Following a head injury, most people will have a mild headache for one to three days. See your doctor for an initial evaluation. If the headache becomes severe, grows progressively worse, or continues longer than expected, medical reevaluation should be obtained *immediately*.

Other warning signs indicating a need for prompt medical attention are:

- unusual drowsiness, especially progressive drowsiness. During the first 24 hours after a head injury, the injured person should be aroused from sleep every two hours. If there is trouble waking the individual, call your doctor *immediately*.

- persistent vomiting

- oozing of blood or fluid from the nose or ears

- uncontrollable twitching or convulsions

- muscle weakness or numbness of the arms and/or legs

- sudden or progressive vision problems

- unexplained fever

WHEN TO BE CONCERNED

How can you tell when your headache requires a doctor's attention? Although the severity of your pain may not be a clue, if it appears suddenly and without reason, especially if you rarely get headaches, you should call your doctor *immediately*. Since tension headaches usually appear during a stressful day, be concerned when a headache wakes you from sleep. A headache that seems to worsen every day despite home treatment is also a cause for concern. Any headache associated with convulsions (*see* Convulsions), dizziness (*see* Dizziness), head injury (*see* Head Injury Precautions), or very high fever (with or without neck stiffness) requires immediate medical evaluation. These symptoms may indicate a serious condition.

TREATMENT

Treatment of your headache depends on its cause. If you suffer from tension headaches, rest, relaxation, and freedom from emotional stress are of primary importance. Try lying in your darkened bedroom with a cool cloth over your forehead and doing deep breathing exercises. Forget your troubles for the moment. A hot bath or gentle massage may help to loosen tight muscles. Nonprescription

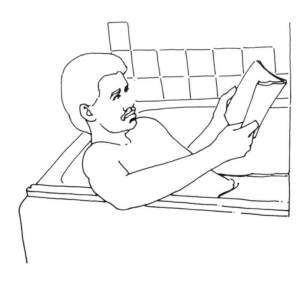

painkillers such as aspirin (if you're not allergic) or acetaminophen may also give relief, but you should never take them for more than a few days. If your headache continues despite home treatment, see your doctor.

If you have classic migraines, your physician may prescribe medication to prevent these attacks. If you are having an acute attack, call your doctor as soon as possible. Treatment is most successful when it is received in the earliest stages of the attack. Your doctor may prescribe a medication that constricts or narrows the blood vessels. Always take these drugs as directed.

If your headache symptoms are the result of any of the other many possible causes, your doctor will first do a thorough evaluation and prescribe appropriate therapy.

CALL YOUR DOCTOR WHEN:

- you suddenly and without reason develop a severe headache, especially if you rarely get headaches.
- your headache worsens every day despite home treatment.
- you have migraine headaches for the first time or you suffer an acute attack.
- your headache wakes you from sleep.
- your headache is associated with convulsions, dizziness, high fever, or a head injury.

Chapter 8

Symptoms and Diseases of the Eyes

BLURRED VISION

DESCRIPTION

The older you get, the greater the chance you will experience some blurring of your vision, because the most common reason for blurred vision is a need for glasses (corrective lenses). People over 40 tend to become farsighted, which means they see better from far away. Small print and things close up tend to appear blurred.

WHEN TO BE CONCERNED

No matter how old you are, if you need glasses, the first symptom you are likely to experience is blurred vision. However, this is not the only cause of this symptom. More serious problems in the eye and diseases that affect the eye include cataracts, glaucoma, detached retina, severe high blood pressure, and diabetes. For that reason, anytime you notice blurring of your vision, you should consult your physician. If your blurring is in only one eye and seems as though a curtain has been thrown over the eye, call your doctor *immediately*. The same is true if your blurred vision is associated with pain, particularly if you've injured your head recently.

TREATMENT

As part of his complete examination, your doctor will test your vision. If you already have glasses or contact lenses, bring them with you. It's possible your blurring may indicate a need for a change in your prescription. Your doctor will also do a special test to check the pressure in your eyes. This determines whether or not you have glaucoma. If you are over 40, you should have your doctor do this test once a year, even if your vision seems perfect. If you have glaucoma, it is important to take the medication your doctor will prescribe since treatment will prevent blindness. If you have one of the other causes of blurred vision, your doctor may need to refer you to an eye specialist, especially if he feels that you may need surgery.

CALL YOUR DOCTOR WHEN:

- you notice gradual blurred vision in both eyes.
- you have painless blurred vision in one eye, like a curtain (*call immediately*).
- your blurred vision is associated with pain and/or head injury (*call immediately*).

BLINDNESS

DESCRIPTION

The gift of sight is something many take for granted. Your eyes are one of your most important and delicate organs. Unless blindness is present at birth or caused by an accident, it almost always comes on gradually. It may result from accidents, chemical or radiation injuries, infections, or brain tumors, among other things. It's difficult to notice small, gradual changes in your vision, but once your vision drops below a certain level, you will finally realize that there's a problem.

Glaucoma is an especially treacherous eye disease that develops gradually and frequently causes blindness. The pressure inside your eye gradually increases and eventually damages the optic nerve leading from the retina of your eye to your brain. Untreated, glaucoma can lead to complete and permanent loss of vision. Though glaucoma may occur in younger people, it is usually seen in people over 40, who commonly experience a gradual loss of peripheral vision. The increased pressure may significantly damage your optic nerve before you are aware of this vision loss.

Poor vision at night, or night blindness, is a vague symptom more common to people in their later years, but any loss of vision may be more apparent at night. Decreased night vision is a symptom of glaucoma and of various other conditions such as cataracts and vitamin A deficiency.

Although they may occur at birth or in young children, cataracts are generally associated with older age and are another possible cause of blindness. A cataract is a clouding of the lens of the eye. The lens ordinarily focuses light from objects onto your retina, and as it becomes cloudy, most images lose their sharp outline. Besides advancing age, diabetes, eye infections, and sudden injuries can also cause cataracts. Nowadays, cataracts are readily treated surgically.

WHEN TO BE CONCERNED

If, despite wearing the proper glasses, you detect a gradual decrease in your vision in one or both eyes, and you are over 40, suspect glaucoma as a possible cause of your symptoms. A loss of peripheral vision and poor night vision may be other signs of glaucoma. Some people also complain of blurred vision as the disease progresses. Others may experience slight pain around the eye or "halos" around lights at night. If you are over 40, routine eye examinations will help to detect glaucoma early.

A gradual and painless loss of vision in someone who is getting on in years may indicate cataracts. Both cataracts and glaucoma cause a gradual loss of vision. Poor vision caused by cataracts can usually be corrected surgically. Unfortunately, loss of vision from glaucoma is usually permanent. A loss of night vision alone, even without other symptoms, still requires a medical evaluation.

TREATMENT

The best way to prevent blindness caused by glaucoma is prevention through early detection. Once you reach age 40, schedule regular eye examinations. If the pressure in your eye is increased, your doctor may prescribe special eyedrops to help drain the fluid from your eye and lower the pressure. He'll follow your condition carefully and record any changes in your vision or any loss of peripheral vision. If the pressure in your eye cannot be controlled with medication, he may recommend surgery to improve the drainage of fluid from your eye. When glaucoma is discovered early, the eye pressure can be controlled and loss of vision can usually be prevented.

The basic treatment for cataracts is surgical removal of the clouded lens. Prior to surgery, your doctor will discuss the various alternatives, such as glasses or contact lenses, to improve your sight after surgery. Recently, new artificial lenses have also been implanted in the eye during surgery with very good results.

If your only symptom is loss of night vision, your treatment will depend on the underlying cause. Generally, there is no treatment for color blindness.

CALL YOUR DOCTOR WHEN:

- you notice a gradual decrease in vision in one or both eyes that is not corrected by new glasses.
- you have any pain in or around your eyeball, you see halos around lights, or you have poor night vision.

SQUINTING OR CROSSED EYES

DESCRIPTION

Each of your eyes is precisely controlled by six small muscles that rotate it in its socket. Normally, these muscles are perfectly balanced so that your eyes focus together. However, a strange symptom called squinting may be present at birth, or it may develop early in childhood. Crossed eyes (strabismus) is another symptom caused by the same underlying problem.

In young children, crossed eyes usually result from weakness or poor coordination of these muscles. When both eyes focus improperly, the brain "hides" or ignores one eye's image to avoid seeing double. Your child may squint to suppress the image from the unfocused eye. The problem is that the eye that is ignored becomes "lazy." If this situation is not detected and treated promptly by age two or three, the "lazy" eye may permanently lose vision.

The development of crossed eyes in adults is usually associated with double vision and double vision is even more significant in adults than in children. Do not ignore even brief periods of double vision without getting a careful medical evaluation. The nerves that control your eye muscles run beneath your brain. Any injury or pressure on these nerves can cause double vision.

WHEN TO BE CONCERNED

If you notice that your child's eyes look crossed or that the child squints occasionally, arrange a prompt eye examination. Don't delay. Remember, after age three, permanent damage can result.

As an adult, if you experience any double vision, even for a short time, you should see your doctor. If you also have associated headaches, dizziness, nausea, vomiting, or blurred vision, a more serious underlying neurological problem may be causing these symptoms. Immediate diagnosis and treatment of the underlying cause is paramount.

TREATMENT

Eyedrops and special glasses may be used to treat a mild imbalance of the eye muscles in early childhood. They force the muscles in each eye to focus evenly. Often surgery is required to correct this imbalance if medical treatment is ineffective. After surgery, your doctor will likely recommend eye exercises to strengthen and coordinate your child's eye muscles.

The treatment of crossed eyes or double vision in an adult depends on the diagnosis and treatment of the underlying cause. Call your doctor when you experience any blurred or double vision even if it is intermittent or temporary.

CALL YOUR DOCTOR WHEN:

- you notice that your child's eyes look crossed or you notice your child squinting.
- you experience any double vision, even if it is temporary and without blurred vision.

EYE TRAUMA

DESCRIPTION

Your eyes are your windows on the world. As one of your most delicate and sensitive organs, they are subject to severe and permanent damage. Most eye injuries fall into two major categories: blunt trauma and foreign body injuries.

Blunt trauma is the kind of injury that results when some outside force or object like a fist or a tennis ball hits your eye. Fortunately, this type of injury doesn't always cause serious damage to your eye since the eye is surrounded and protected by its bony socket. Sometimes, however, tissues surrounding the eye are bruised, leaving you with a black eye.

It is also possible that the force of such an injury can cause your retina to loosen and actually peel away (detached retina). This may be associated with bleeding inside the eye. A sudden change in your vision, as well as the pain that occurs, will generally alert you to these problems. Occasionally, the lens of your eye may also be dislocated. A more alarming but far less serious injury is a small hemorrhage (subconjunctival hemorrhage) (see Bloodshot Eye) that occurs under the skin of the eyeball.

A more common type of eye injury occurs when a foreign body enters your eye. This foreign body can be anything from an eyelash to a speck of dirt or dust to a dangerous chemical like battery acid. Such injuries are usually very painful because they irritate your cornea, which is extremely sensitive. Some of these injuries are real medical emergencies requiring immediate treatment to prevent blindness.

WHEN TO BE CONCERNED

A blunt injury to your eye that results in any loss of vision or double vision is a medical emergency. Suspect a possible retinal detachment. Your retina is the sensitive layer of nerve fibers behind the eye that receives light and transmits the image to your brain. When your retina is torn or detached, the most common symptom is a veil or curtain that clouds your vision. This may be caused by damage to your retina or bleeding into your eye. Both of these conditions require *immediate* medical attention.

If you suddenly feel a particle in your eye, such as an eyelash, a small insect, or a speck of soot, carefully try to remove it *immediately*. If you can't flush it out easily with clean water and a moistened swab, or if you have persistent pain, see your doctor promptly. Foreign bodies in the eye often cause corneal abrasions, infections, and, in a few cases, even perforations of the cornea.

TREATMENT

Following a blunt injury and a loss of vision, lie on your back as quickly as possible and avoid any unnecessary movement. Sudden movements will aggravate any injury to your retina or bleeding into your eye. Once you've suffered a loss of vision, there is no home treatment except for cold packs to relieve any swelling around your eye while you are on your way to the emergency room. Don't drive! Have someone take you to a properly equipped hospital *immediately*. Your doctor will probably consult a specialist in ophthalmology to help evaluate and treat your symptoms.

There are a few good techniques for promptly removing a small particle from your eye. First, try simply flushing your eye with large amounts of water. This alone often removes an eyelash, a loose particle, or a small insect that has gotten into your eye. If the particle is trapped under your upper lid, try drawing the lid down over your lower lid several times. Often this will remove the particle.

Don't rub your eye or eyelids. Your cornea is the very sensitive clear central area of your eye. Any pressure on your eye or eyelid may embed the particle in your cornea or scratch its delicate surface. Your cornea is thin and clear, and it has no blood supply. It is easily infected, and it may perforate easily, with the infection spreading into the eye. Any persistent speck in the eye or suspected corneal injury requires prompt medical treatment.

CALL YOUR DOCTOR WHEN:

- you have any loss of vision or double vision following blunt trauma to your eye.
- you cannot easily remove any foreign body from your eye.
- you have any pain or decrease in vision after a foreign body has been removed.
- you have any chemical injury to your eye (call immediately).

BLOODSHOT EYE

DESCRIPTION

Because the tissues in your eye are so delicate and so close together, it will often be difficult for you to distinguish one symptom from another. A good example of this difficulty is the symptom that most people call a "bloodshot eye." There are several possible causes for redness or irritation on the white portion of the eyeball.

The most common cause of this symptom is an inflammation of the thin skin (conjunctiva) that covers the eyeball and lines the eyelids. This condition is commonly known as "pink eye" (conjunctivitis). It may be caused by a bacterial or viral infection or by any irritating substance such as smoke or suntan lotion.

When you have conjunctivitis, your eye will water and your eyeball will become bloodshot. When the cause is a viral infection, your eye will usually look pink. If you have a bacterial conjunctivitis, your eye will appear red and angry-looking. There may be a yellowish pus discharge, and, in severe cases, your eyelids may become swollen. Your vision may even be temporarily blurred.

Another common cause of redness in your eye is a small hemorrhage under the thin skin that covers your eyeball. This results from a rupture or break in one of the small blood vessels on the surface of your eye. These small hemorrhages may follow a mild eye injury or even a sneeze or a cough. They may take two or three weeks to clear up completely, and they usually have no effect on your vision. In fact, unless you look in the mirror or your friends tell you about it, you won't even know you have a subconjunctival hemorrhage.

A third cause of a red or pink eye that generally is much more serious is a condition known as iritis. If you have iritis, the colored part of your eye (iris) will be inflamed. As the condition worsens, your pain will become more severe and may travel to the side of your head. The white portion of your eye around the cornea may become red, and your vision may blur.

Iritis usually involves only one eye, but it may involve both eyes at the same time. As this condition progresses, tearing and light sensitivity may develop. In the later stages, any movement of the eye may be painful.

WHEN TO BE CONCERNED

Generally, there is no danger to your vision from mild conjunctivitis. Severe bacterial infections with pus and drainage can be quite uncomfortable and occasionally may spread to other areas of the eye, causing serious problems. Also, many types of eye infections are contagious, so avoid direct contact with others. If you suspect that you have a bacterial conjunctivitis, or if the condition persists for more than two or three days, get prompt medical attention. Any loss of vision requires *immediate* medical evaluation.

Generally, a small bright red area of blood on the white portion of your eye should not be a cause for alarm. If your vision is normal and there is no pain, you probably don't need immediate medical attention. However, if you notice more than one of these hemorrhages, or both eyes are affected, and/or there is pain or decreased vision, see your doctor promptly.

When you have the symptom of a bloodshot eye along with pain deep in your eyeball, you should suspect iritis. If your pain persists, your vision becomes blurred, or your eye becomes extremely sensitive to light, seek *immediate* medical attention. If not treated properly, iritis can permanently damage your eye.

TREATMENT

If you have mild conjunctivitis caused by a virus or an irritant such as smoke, and your vision is normal, warm compresses may help to relieve your mild discomfort. Wear sunglasses to prevent any irritation and spasm caused by bright sunlight. Keep your eye clean and be careful not to spread any infection. If your symptoms are more severe or last longer than two or three days, see your doctor. He may take a culture from the drainage and prescribe antibiotic drops. In some cases, if he suspects that your symptoms stem from an allergy, he may prescribe cortisone drops.

There is generally no required treatment for a simple subconjunctival hemorrhage. Avoid any strenuous activity and be certain that it begins to resolve within a few days. See your doctor if your vision changes or the small hemorrhage persists. He will evaluate your symptoms to be sure that there is no serious underlying cause.

There is no home treatment for iritis. If you suspect this condition at all, see your doctor *immediately*. He may use a special microscope, called a slit lamp, to examine your eye. If you do have iritis, you'll probably require prescription medication. Your doctor may also recommend steroid therapy and try to find an underlying cause. Iritis can result in loss of vision if it is not treated promptly and followed up with medical supervision.

CALL YOUR DOCTOR WHEN:

- you have a red or bloodshot eye that persists for more than two or three days.
- you have a bloodshot eye with a thick yellowish discharge.
- you have a small hemorrhage on the surface of your eye that does not go away in one or two weeks.
- you have more than one small eye hemorrhage.
- your eye is red and you have pain or blurred vision.

Chapter 9

Symptoms and Diseases of the Ears, Nose, and Throat

BLEEDING OR DISCHARGE FROM THE EAR

DESCRIPTION

If you have bleeding or discharge of any material from your ear, you are not likely to overlook these symptoms. Besides the discharge itself, you will probably experience pain from the irritation of the sensitive skin in your ear canal (*see* Earache) and even a noticeable hearing loss in the involved ear (*see* Hearing Loss and Deafness).

Your eardrum is a thin membrane separating the external ear canal from the delicate structures of the middle ear. When your middle ear is infected, the eardrum may become reddened and bulge outward. If the eardrum suddenly ruptures (perforates), blood and/or yellow pus-filled fluid may drain from the canal. Pain and hearing loss are associated symptoms. Voices may sound hollow, and you may feel dizzy. The bleeding, however, from a perforated eardrum will usually be minimal.

Bleeding from the ear can occur following a severe head injury. Typically, there will be other associated symptoms such as blurred or double vision, nausea, vomiting, and even possible loss of consciousness.

While most yellow discharges result from middle ear infections, a boil or other infection in your ear canal may produce the same symptom. If you have a large enough boil, you may also experience a full feeling in the ear and possibly decreased hearing due to swelling and blockage of the canal.

Other infections in your external ear canal may cause itching as well as discharge. If the infection is due to bacteria, the discharge will be yellow, but if it is caused by a fungus, it may appear grayish-white or black. Fungal infections are often the result of swimming in contaminated water and/or poor hygiene and usually cause more discharge and itching than actual pain.

If you have had a head injury, a watery discharge from your ear may indicate that spinal fluid is leaking from a skull fracture. Get *immediate* medical attention. *This is an emergency.*

WHEN TO BE CONCERNED

Any bleeding from the ear, whether it is associated with pain or a head or ear trauma, should be a cause for concern and requires prompt medical evaluation. Likewise, if you notice a watery discharge following any head injury, seek *immediate* medical attention. Your doctor will diagnose and treat the underlying condition. If the bleeding or discharge resulted from head trauma, you'll need a thorough neurological evaluation.

Bleeding from a perforated eardrum also requires appropriate therapy. Untreated middle ear infections can lead to serious complications, including meningitis and inflammation of the bone behind your ear (mastoiditis). Mastoiditis itself can cause a thick, yellow discharge from the ear and severe pain.

Generally, any discharge from your ear should be checked by your doctor.

TREATMENT

There is no home treatment for bleeding or a discharge from your ear. See your doctor as soon as possible to determine the underlying cause. In the meantime, keep your ear clean and dry and simply cover it with a light gauze dressing. Don't attempt to wash or drain it since, with a perforated eardrum, this can lead to a serious ear infection. Do not put anything, including cotton-tipped applicators, in your ear.

If you've suffered any head or ear injury, your doctor will take an especially careful history. He'll clean your ear canal and try to determine the underlying cause of your bleeding or discharge. If he suspects a skull injury or involvement of the mastoid bone, he will order special X-rays. If bleeding stems from a simple perforation, he may prescribe antibiotics to prevent infection. If your doctor finds a boil or other infection in the canal, he may get a culture to determine the cause and prescribe the appropriate antibiotics.

CALL YOUR DOCTOR WHEN:

- you notice any blood or watery liquid coming from your ear canal, even without a history of head injury.
- you have a thick yellowish or grayish-white discharge from your ear.

EAR INFECTIONS

DESCRIPTION

Any infection of your ear is called otitis. External otitis means that the infection is in your ear canal, while otitis media means the infection is in the middle ear.

If you have external otitis, you may experience itching, pain, a discharge from your ear, and/or a hearing loss. If you have allergies, you may be particularly susceptible to this type of infection. This is especially true anytime you let your ears get wet, such as when swimming or when you use an irritant around your ears such as hair spray or hair dye. If you try to clean the earwax from your ears too vigorously or scratch an itching ear with dirty hands, you may also develop external otitis.

Middle ear infections may be either acute or chronic. Acute otitis media is most common in infants and children but may occur at any age. Often otitis media accompanies or follows a nose or throat infection. The germs causing the infection (either bacteria or viruses) travel to the middle ear through a tube that connects the middle ear to the throat (eustachian tube).

Typically, you will experience ear pain, fever, decreased hearing, and a feeling of pressure or fullness in the ear. Infants and children often have other associated symptoms, such as loss of appetite, vomiting, diarrhea, or sleepiness. If they aren't talking yet, they may just pull at the infected ear. If the eardrum suddenly ruptures (perforates), bloody and/or pus-filled fluid may drain from your ear (see Bleeding or Discharge from the Ear). When the perforation is permanent (as determined by physician), chronic infection develops.

WHEN TO BE CONCERNED

External otitis is generally not serious and will resolve quickly with treatment. Middle ear infections, if untreated, can lead to serious complications, including meningitis, inflammation of the bone behind your ear (mastoiditis), perforation of the eardrum with chronic infection and/or permanent hearing loss (see Hearing Loss and Deafness). Anytime you have a severe earache, see your doctor to prevent these problems.

TREATMENT

If you have an ear infection, your doctor will need to examine your ears and determine the location of the infection. He may suggest avoiding air travel until your condition improves. If you have external otitis, he will probably prescribe eardrops containing antibiotics and/or steroids after taking a culture. Follow his instructions carefully and remember to keep water away from your ears during treatment.

If you have a middle ear infection, your physician will probably prescribe oral antibiotics (if it is caused by bacteria) and possibly decongestants and pain medication. If the infection does not resolve promptly with this treatment, or when bulging of the eardrum indicates that a discharge is present and under pressure, he may need to make a small opening in the eardrum (myringotomy) to allow drainage. The eardrum usually heals naturally.

If you have chronic otitis media associated with a perforated eardrum, the hole can generally be repaired. Your doctor will refer you to a specialist in ear surgery.

CALL YOUR DOCTOR WHEN:

- you or your child has a severe earache with or without other symptoms.

EARACHE

DESCRIPTION

Your ears are extremely sensitive, so even mild irritation of your earlobe and outer ear canal can hurt as much as or more than a severe middle ear infection. Certain nerves that supply pain fibers to your ear also supply other areas around your face, so your ear may ache in the absence of ear disease. This is called referred pain and can be the result of problems in your nose, sinuses, teeth, gums, jaw, tongue, tonsils, voice box (larynx), windpipe (trachea), or food tube (esophagus). Tumors in these locations may first make their presence known by pain referred to your ear.

WHEN TO BE CONCERNED

Because ear pain can represent problems inside or outside your ear, you should always consult a physician when your pain is severe and persistent, whether your hearing is affected or not. Anytime you notice blood coming from your ear (*see* Bleeding or Discharge from the Ear) or you have had a head injury, seek *immediate* medical attention. The most common cause of earache in children is middle ear infection. This requires prompt examination and treatment by a physician to prevent serious complications.

TREATMENT

To treat an earache, the cause must be identified and treated appropriately. If you have an infection on your earlobe, the soft skin of the lobe may throb and appear red and warm. Typically, this is the result of a pimple on the skin or a reaction from pierced ears. Try applying warm compresses (a hot, clean washcloth on the lobe for 5-15 minutes three times a day), but never squeeze any pimple. Remove your earrings and don't wear them again until the irritation has resolved. If you are allergic to the metal in the earrings, buy only hypoallergenic earrings. Whenever the symptom doesn't go away within a day or two, see your doctor.

Irritation in the inner part of the canal may be accompanied by itching. Your doctor will want to examine the canal and, if necessary, prescribe eardrops. If you have a middle ear infection (*see* Ear Infections), he will prescribe antibiotics and possibly medication to relieve the pain.

CALL YOUR DOCTOR WHEN:

• you have a severe or persistent earache.

HEARING LOSS AND DEAFNESS

DESCRIPTION

You may experience hearing loss at any age. How disabled you will be depends on the degree of your loss, your age (whether you've already learned to talk), and whether one or both ears are affected. About 5-10 percent of people have some temporary or permanent hearing loss severe enough to disrupt their normal function.

Children may be born with impaired hearing as a result of failure of the ear to form properly, infections in the mother during pregnancy (such as German measles and influenza), or injuries during birth itself. Childhood diseases like mumps and middle ear infections may produce hearing loss. Other causes include high doses of drugs such as aspirin, injuries to the ear, excessive earwax (*see* Impacted Earwax), and tumors. A rare disease called Ménière's produces periodic attacks of hearing loss, usually only in one ear, associated with nausea, vomiting, vertigo, and sweating.

Teenagers exposed to repeated loud music will likely notice some hearing loss as they get older in addition to the decreased hearing that everyone notices with aging.

WHEN TO BE CONCERNED

Alert parents can often detect hearing loss in young infants (six to nine months) by their failure to respond to appropriate sounds. If your child was premature, the birth was difficult, or you (the mother) had a viral infection during pregnancy, your child may have a higher risk of hearing loss than other children. Whenever your child isn't learning to talk the way he should, seems unable to concentrate, or is slow in learning, have your doctor check him for a possible hearing problem.

Likewise, see your doctor if you notice a hearing loss in yourself, especially if it is sudden and/or associated with a head injury, discharge from your ear (*see* Bleeding or Discharge from the Ear), earache (*see* Earache), or ringing in the ears (*see* Ringing in the Ears).

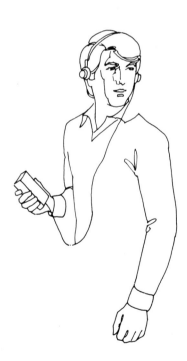

TREATMENT

A complete ear, nose, and throat exam is essential for anyone with the symptom of hearing loss. Your doctor will check the ear canal, eardrum, and middle ear to detect even slight abnormalities that might be causing your problem. He may also need to do special hearing tests. Be sure to let your doctor know if you are taking any medication, including aspirin, since that could be the cause of your hearing problem.

If your hearing loss is caused by noise, sometimes avoiding loud noises for about six months will improve your hearing. You can prevent this kind of hearing loss by wearing earplugs or other noise attenuators whenever you must be in a noisy environment and by not listening to amplified music.

If you or your child has an ear infection (*see* Ear Infections), prompt treatment will generally restore hearing to normal. Any damage to your eardrum or any of the structures in the middle ear may be repaired surgically. If your doctor determines that the hearing loss is not correctable, he may recommend a hearing aid. Young children may need speech therapy.

CALL YOUR DOCTOR WHEN:

- you suspect a hearing loss in your child.
- you have a hearing loss.

IMPACTED EARWAX

DESCRIPTION

The glands of the outer part of your ear secrete a sticky yellow-brown substance called cerumen (earwax) that protects the delicate skin lining your ear canal. Normally, the wax dries and falls out of the ear. However, when it gets packed deep in the canal (usually due to your repeated unskilled attempts to remove it), the wax becomes impacted and actually blocks the ear passage. You may experience a feeling of fullness, deafness (*see* Hearing Loss and Deafness), or ringing in the ears (*see* Ringing in the Ears).

WHEN TO BE CONCERNED

Impacted cerumen is not serious, but it can affect your hearing, and removing it yourself improperly could injure the eardrum.

TREATMENT

You have probably been warned not to put anything bigger than your elbow in your ear. In a sense, that's no joke. Any time you try to remove earwax from your ear canal, unless you do it properly and gently, you run the risk of injuring your eardrum. If the wax is easily movable, you can insert a cotton-tipped swab just inside the canal and pull it out with a gentle rolling motion.

If the wax is too hard, you can purchase softening drops (carbamide peroxide in anhydrous glycerol) at your pharmacy. Put two to three drops in each ear, two or three times a day for two or three days. Be aware, however, these drops can sometimes cause an irritation, so check with your doctor before using them. Once the wax is soft, it is usually easy to remove it gently with a swab. If the wax has become impacted and you can't remove it yourself, consult your physician. He may use a curette or irrigation with warm water.

CALL YOUR DOCTOR WHEN:

- you have earwax that is too hard or too deep in the canal to remove easily.

NOSEBLEED

DESCRIPTION

Nosebleeds (epistaxes) can be alarming, but they occur commonly and often are not serious. They are frequent in childhood, especially after blunt trauma and with colds and hay fever involving severe sneezing. More severe nosebleeds are common in older people as a result of hardening of the arteries and high blood pressure. Other causes include growths in the nose, certain diseases, and nose picking.

Most nosebleeds begin suddenly and without warning. Although there is rarely a significant blood loss, the bleeding may seem considerable. It usually comes from a network of veins just inside your nostrils, but, in more severe cases, it may come from arteries farther back in your nose.

WHEN TO BE CONCERNED

Bleeding that comes from the small veins just inside your nose usually stops promptly when you apply pressure. More profuse and prolonged bleeding comes from arteries farther back in the nose and is more commonly caused by hypertension, requiring prompt medical attention.

Generally, you should be concerned when your nosebleed persists or recurs without an obvious cause. See your doctor promptly to stop the bleeding and find the underlying cause. Severe nosebleeds may also be associated with liver disease, blood disorders, or tumors of the nasal sinuses.

TREATMENT

To treat a simple nosebleed at home, insert a small sterile cotton plug into each nostril and pinch them together firmly between your thumb and forefinger for 5-10 minutes. Try to relax. Sit quietly but don't lie down. Avoid swallowing blood and spit it out if it collects in the back of your throat. After 5-6 minutes, gradually release the pressure on your nostrils and see if your nosebleed has stopped. If it cannot be controlled by this simple procedure, or if it recurs, see your doctor promptly to be sure that a more serious condition is not causing this symptom.

In severe cases, when arteries farther back in your nose are involved, a doctor will need to tightly pack this area to control bleeding. In extreme cases, these arteries may need to be tied off surgically. These more serious nosebleeds are much more common in older people and those with high blood pressure.

CALL YOUR DOCTOR WHEN:

- you have a nosebleed that keeps recurring after 30-60 minutes.
- your nosebleed recurs more than once or twice.

POSTNASAL DRIP

DESCRIPTION

This common symptom is usually caused by increased mucus production from the lining of the nasal membranes. Another common cause is sinusitis due to allergy. There is usually a constant nasal discharge, and much of this mucus may drain down your throat. This drainage often causes a chronic cough and occasionally may cause a choking sensation. If your postnasal discharge is chronic, you may also find that you have bad breath (halitosis).

WHEN TO BE CONCERNED

If you are suffering from a chronic postnasal drip that is not associated with an acute cold or other respiratory infection, seek a medical evaluation to determine the underlying cause. Hay fever or another allergy may contribute to your symptoms. Other symptoms associated with an allergic condition include itchy, watery eyes and sneezing. If your voice has changed and taken on a nasal quality, be concerned about a possible growth in one of your sinuses or behind your nose (nasopharynx). If your nasal discharge is tinged with blood, see your doctor promptly.

TREATMENT

Treatment of postnasal discharge basically consists of treatment of the underlying cause. Postnasal drainage due to an acute respiratory infection will quickly clear up with your other symptoms. Home treatment for your cold itself (*see* Cold) will usually be all that is necessary. If your symptoms stem from a chronic allergic condition and they are especially bothersome, your doctor will try to determine the cause of your allergy and recommend appropriate treatment or desensitization.

If your postnasal drip has come on suddenly, you may try a short course of decongestants. Be careful to avoid the prolonged use of decongestants or antihistamines.

CALL YOUR DOCTOR WHEN:

- you have a postnasal drip that is persistent and not associated with a cold or an allergy that is already being treated.
- you notice a change or a nasal quality in your voice.
- you notice that your nasal drainage is blood-tinged or pinkish.

COLD

DESCRIPTION

The "common cold" is indeed just that—common. This ailment very likely affects mankind more frequently than any other. It may be caused by literally dozens of different viruses. Because of this, an adequate vaccine in the near future is unlikely, and you can expect recurrences since you are unlikely to develop immunity. Many of these different viruses can also be found in healthy people in the absence of cold symptoms.

Other symptoms often associated with the characteristic nasal mucus drainage and stuffiness include tiredness, muscle aches and pains, headache, and a low-grade fever. The mucous membranes in your nose usually become reddened and swollen, and your throat and tonsils may also become red and swollen. The glands in your neck may become slightly enlarged and tender.

Most colds are spread by droplets from coughing or sneezing, and the incubation period is usually between one and four days. If you are in generally good health, you're still likely to catch a cold from time to time. If you are run-down, you are generally more susceptible. Despite the many old wives' tales you've heard, there is no clear evidence that cold or dampness contributes to the common cold.

WHEN TO BE CONCERNED

While your symptoms will usually last for only a few days without any other complications, occasionally other problems may develop. These complications are usually due to secondary bacterial infections that result from your run-down condition. If you develop a high fever or a thick yellowish nasal drainage, suspect a sinus infection (*see* Sinusitis). Severe ear pain with or without drainage from your ear and decreased hearing suggest the possibility of an ear infection (*see* Ear Infections). A high fever, a cough, and heavy yellow sputum production are symptoms of pneumonia (*see* Cough). Finally, a severe sore throat with swollen neck glands (lymph nodes) suggests bacterial tonsillitis (*see* Sore Throat). If your headache becomes severe or you develop neck stiffness, you require *immediate* medical evaluation.

Whenever you have a cold and develop a high fever (over 102 degrees Fahrenheit), or whenever you develop any of the above symptoms, seek prompt medical attention. Often, bacteria that are normally in your nose and throat cause these other serious illnesses as a result of your weakened defenses. These complications are even more common in young children and the elderly because of their generally poorer resistance. If you have a serious chronic illness such as diabetes, heart or lung disease, or a blood disorder, you should probably see your doctor even for symptoms of a cold.

TREATMENT

There is still no specific treatment available for the common cold. Despite what you may think, antibiotics are effective only in treating complicating bacterial infections. Treating yourself at home will almost always be as effective as visiting your doctor unless you suspect a complication.

Generally, you should get plenty of rest, lots of fluid, and a balanced diet. You may take aspirin (unless you are allergic to it; children should not be given aspirin) for headaches, sore throat, muscle aches, or fever, but be careful to avoid masking other complications with too much medication to relieve your symptoms. In general, except for a mild expectorant to help break up your phlegm or a mild decongestant, you should avoid heavy use of over-the-counter preparations and let nature take its course. To relieve a sore throat, you can try warm saltwater gargles, and steam inhalation may help to relieve your cough and nasal congestion.

CALL YOUR DOCTOR WHEN:

• you have cold symptoms that persist or you have a chronic illness that may make you more susceptible to complications.

- you develop a high fever (over 102 degrees Fahrenheit) with or without symptoms of other complications.
- you develop symptoms that suggest a complication such as tonsillitis, pneumonia, sinusitis, or ear infection (*call immediately*).

SINUSITIS

DESCRIPTION

Your sinuses are air spaces in your skull that are lined with mucous membranes and give a normal quality to your voice. These sinuses also play a role in warming, moistening, and filtering the air you breathe. Even under normal circumstances, your sinuses drain poorly, and when mucous secretions build up, the drainage usually gets even worse. When this occurs, headaches and congestion usually follow. When sinusitis is caused by bacterial infection, symptoms include a fever, moderate to severe pain over your sinuses, and a thick yellowish drainage that contains pus.

This bacterial infection may develop from a simple cold, nasal polyps, or allergies. Various types of bacteria cause these infections, and the normally poor drainage can make treatment difficult. The main symptom of severe sinusitis is headache with pain on both sides of the nose and around your eyes. When a bacterial sinusitis becomes chronic, the mucous membranes lining your sinuses become thickened and swollen.

WHEN TO BE CONCERNED

If yellowish mucus persists for more than a day or two, seek prompt medical attention. You should realize that most serious cases of sinusitis are caused by a bacterial infection and generally do require a medical evaluation and treatment with antibiotics.

If you develop headache and tenderness over your sinuses following a simple cold or allergic rhinitis, or nasal inflammation, suspect bacterial sinusitis. A fever and a thick yellowish discharge should serve to confirm your suspicions. The amount of blockage will determine the sinus tenderness and headache that you experience. If sinusitis is not treated promptly, you may develop other complications such as bronchitis, pneumonia, ear infections, and even meningitis.

Finally, acute sinusitis that has become severe may cause both fever and chills, loss of smell (anosmia), drowsiness, dizziness, and swelling around your eyes. These symptoms require *immediate* medical attention.

TREATMENT

If your sinusitis is mild and caused by a virus, your only home treatment will be warm compresses over the sinuses, decongestants, and aspirin (if you have no allergy). Generally, avoid antihistamines, which can dry out your mucous membranes and worsen your problem.

Strangely, if your condition is more serious and due to a bacterial infection, more effective treatment is available. Your doctor will probably get a culture of your secretions and prescribe antibiotics. He may also recommend application of heat over your infected sinuses as well as various procedures to aid in drainage of the pus. The most common complication of acute sinusitis is chronic sinusitis. Once a sinus infection becomes chronic, its management becomes more difficult. Often your sinuses will need to be drained repeatedly. With any sinus infection, you should blow your nose carefully and absolutely avoid smoking.

CALL YOUR DOCTOR WHEN:

- you develop persistent sinus drainage that follows a cold or allergy and lasts longer than two or three days.
- you develop a fever and/or pain over your sinuses with or without a thick yellowish discharge.
- you develop a loss of smell, drowsiness, dizziness, or swelling around your eyes (*call immediately*).

ALLERGIC RHINITIS

DESCRIPTION

Nasal drainage is a common symptom associated with allergies. If you suffer from hay fever, you are familiar with the endless watery nasal discharge, the sneezing, and the itchy eyes. All of these symptoms are part of your body's allergic response to a foreign substance such as pollen, molds, or fungus spores. When this occurs, the membranes in your nasal passages become swollen. Certain white blood cells (eosinophiles) present in your mucous secretions will strongly indicate to your doctor the possibility of an allergic basis for your symptoms.

WHEN TO BE CONCERNED

Allergic rhinitis is an uncomfortable condition although it is usually not a cause for serious concern. Most acute attacks are self-limited, and the symptoms can usually be relieved with antihista-mines. Be very concerned if you also experience a generalized allergic reaction with asthmatic-type symptoms of wheezing and shortness of breath.

TREATMENT

A short course of antihistamines is the mainstay of home treatment for allergic rhinitis. It is important that you avoid taking these medications for longer than a few days since they may overly dry your mucous membranes. Also, avoid topical or local decongestants since they can aggravate or perpetuate chronic rhinitis. Try to determine the source of your allergy. You may be especially allergic to a particular type of pollen, dander from a house pet, a particular piece of furniture or carpet, or even house dust. Dustproof masks or home air filters may help to remove offending substances from the air you breathe.

In more severe attacks, your doctor may suggest adrenaline-type drugs in combination with antihistamines. If your symptoms still can't be controlled, he may even recommend steroid medications for a few days until you are feeling better. These medications should be discontinued as soon as possible. Finally, your doctor may suggest allergy testing to identify the particular allergen causing your symptoms. If one can be identified, a program of gradual desensitization with the allergen may be effective.

CALL YOUR DOCTOR WHEN:

- you have a chronic watery nasal discharge with or without itchy, watery eyes.
- you have other associated allergic symptoms such as wheezing or shortness of breath.

BAD BREATH

DESCRIPTION

Although most people consider bad breath to be a social problem, it may actually be a symptom of a more serious disorder. It is most commonly caused by foods such as onions or garlic. A less obvious but especially common cause in the elderly is infected gums and poorly fitting dentures. Smoking also commonly causes bad breath.

There are also some unusual but far more serious causes of this symptom. Chronic infections of the sinuses (*see* Sinusitis), mouth, throat, and lungs often cause a foul odor. Heavy smokers with chronic bronchitis, lung abscesses, or lung cancer also often have bad breath. Similarly, infections and tumors of the digestive organs cause foul-smelling breath.

WHEN TO BE CONCERNED

If you have developed this symptom, look for a serious underlying cause. Begin with a thorough dental examination, in which your dentist will look for poor oral hygiene, gum infections, poorly fitting dentures, or dental abscesses. If you still can't find a likely cause, schedule a medical evaluation. Give your doctor a careful medical history. Are you a smoker? Do you have a chronic cough? Do you have bleeding gums or a gastrointestinal problem? Do you vomit or have indigestion frequently? Have you lost weight recently? All of these answers may help your physician find the underlying cause of your problem.

TREATMENT

The treatment of bad breath depends on the underlying cause. Besides certain foods, poor oral hygiene is the usual culprit. Obviously, your home treatment should focus on good dental hygiene. Try regular brushing, dental floss, and possibly a water pick to remove food particles from between your teeth. Cases caused by serious, chronic infections or tumors in the respiratory or gastrointestinal system require careful diagnosis and treatment.

CALL YOUR DOCTOR WHEN:

- your bad breath has persisted for two or three weeks despite good oral hygiene.
- you have bad breath associated with a chronic gum infection or poorly fitting dentures.
- you have bad breath associated with a chronic cough, indigestion, or weight loss.

BLEEDING GUMS

DESCRIPTION

Bleeding gums are rarely a serious symptom, but occasionally they may suggest a major underlying illness. Simply brushing too vigorously with a stiff-bristled toothbrush may be the cause. If so, your bleeding should stop quickly. Localized mouth infections such as trench mouth, which inflame your gums, also often cause bleeding. Your gums will be sore and bleed repeatedly at the slightest touch. Certain rare diseases such as scurvy and pellegra, caused by vitamin deficiencies, often caused bleeding gums in the past.

But the most serious underlying condition that causes repeated bleeding is a generalized blood disorder. Often bleeding gums will be the first sign of a blood clotting disorder. Various types of anemia, hemophilia, vitamin C or K deficiency, or leukemia may cause these problems.

WHEN TO BE CONCERNED

Don't be alarmed if your gums bleed only once in a while after vigorous brushing or using dental floss. This is normal. If, on the other hand, your gums are chronically swollen and tender and ooze blood at the slightest touch, suspect a gum infection. See your dentist first to check for gum disease. Various infections or problems caused by a vitamin deficiency have a characteristic appearance.

If your gums bleed regularly, and you have no signs of gum disease or a vitamin deficiency, other serious causes need to be ruled out. Your doctor will take a careful medical history and order certain routine blood tests to be sure your blood clots properly. If you have other signs of abnormal bleeding such as bruising easily (*see* Bleeding or Abnormal Bruising) or blood in your stool or urine, you should be especially concerned and seek *immediate* medical attention.

TREATMENT

Occasional bleeding of your gums following vigorous brushing does not require treatment. A dental specialist should treat most gum infections. If your problem is a generalized bleeding disorder, you'll need an immediate medical evaluation and specialized treatment, depending on your underlying condition.

CALL YOUR DOCTOR WHEN:

- you have chronic bleeding or blood oozing from tender, inflamed gums.
- your gums bleed regularly at the slightest touch or for no reason at all.
- your gums bleed and you have other symptoms of bleeding or you bruise easily.

SORE THROAT

DESCRIPTION

A sore throat is a general symptom that simply describes an inflammation of the mucous membranes lining the area around the base of your tongue and your tonsils. Any number of illnesses can cause this area to become red, swollen, and painful. Usually, your sore throat will be just one of the symptoms associated with an acute viral illness such as a common cold or flu. You may experience nasal and sinus congestion, a cough, low-grade fever, and swollen glands as well.

Another common viral illness that often begins with symptoms of a severe sore throat is mononucleosis. This highly contagious condition is usually more serious and prolonged than a simple cold and often involves your liver and spleen as well as causing characteristic changes in your blood cells. Other symptoms associated with this condition include a generalized rash and extreme tiredness. Mononucleosis is transmitted in saliva, and for this reason it is commonly known as the "kissing disease."

It is generally important to determine whether your sore throat is caused by a virus like cold or flu or a bacterial infection, most commonly "strep" (streptococcus infection). The term tonsillitis is usually used to describe a bacterial infection. Although a bacterial tonsillitis may occur in any age group, "strep throat" is most common in children. Other bacterial causes of tonsillitis, such as gonorrhea and staph (staphylococcus infection), are more common in adults.

Tonsillitis caused by a bacterial infection usually comes on suddenly and is associated with fever (sometimes as high as 102 degrees Fahrenheit), chills, headache, and swollen neck glands. A throat culture taken by your doctor will usually confirm the diagnosis.

Another type of infection that causes symptoms of a sore throat is a fungus called thrush (Candida albicans) (*see* Irritations of the Mucous Membranes). This condition is most common in infants while bottle-feeding. In adults, this usually occurs in denture wearers or after long-term antibiotic therapy. Since thrush appears in about one-third of normal mouths, an overgrowth of this fungus is common in people with chronic and debilitating diseases such as diabetes or cancer.

Suspect thrush if you see creamy white curdlike patches over your throat and gums. The underlying mucous membranes may be red and swollen and bleed easily. Unlike most other causes of a sore throat, with thrush you will probably not have a fever or swollen neck glands.

WHEN TO BE CONCERNED

If you have a mild sore throat associated with other symptoms of a viral illness, don't worry. Your sore throat will almost always go away in a few days along with your other symptoms. If your sore throat is associated with a high fever (over 102 degrees Fahrenheit), markedly swollen glands, severe headache, or extreme tiredness, suspect bacterial tonsillitis or mononucleosis and promptly consult your doctor.

Extreme tiredness along with these other symptoms suggests mononucleosis as a likely diagnosis. Your doctor will probably suggest a throat culture and possibly a routine blood test to confirm his diagnosis of bacterial tonsillitis or mononucleosis.

If you have whitish curdlike patches in your mouth along with your sore throat, suspect thrush. This condition itself should not cause concern, but because it usually occurs in debilitated adults, see your doctor promptly to rule out a serious underlying cause.

TREATMENT

If your sore throat is caused by a cold or flu virus, it is usually less serious than a bacterial tonsillitis or thrush. A viral sore throat is best treated at home with warm saltwater gargles, rest, and aspirin (if you are not allergic). *Avoid giving aspirin to your children for any viral infection.*

Bacterial tonsillitis usually requires medical diagnosis and treatment with an antibiotic. Your doctor may get a throat culture to confirm his diagnosis before prescribing antibiotics. Be sure to tell him if you are allergic to penicillin or any other medication. Also be sure to take your medication for the full time it is prescribed to prevent complications.

No specific treatment is available for mononucleosis. With this condition, expect to be at complete rest for at least two to four weeks and possibly longer. Your doctor will suggest warm saltwater gargles for your sore throat, aspirin, and an adequate diet. In severe cases, a short course of steroid medications may be recommended. Symptoms of mononucleosis may last as long as three months in severe cases.

Thrush is generally treated every few hours with mouth rinses of equal parts of peroxide and salt solution to relieve the pain and promote healing. A drug called Nystatin, available only by prescription, is also used three times a day as a mouth rinse.

CALL YOUR DOCTOR WHEN:

- you have a sore throat that persists for more than two or three days without other symptoms of a cold or flu.
- your sore throat causes a fever of 102 degrees Fahrenheit or higher and is associated with swollen and tender neck glands.
- you have extreme tiredness associated with a fever and sore throat.
- you have a sore throat with patches of a creamy, white curdlike growth on your throat and gums.

HOARSENESS

DESCRIPTION

Hoarseness is usually a trivial symptom that occasionally indicates a very serious underlying condition. If your symptom is trivial, it will usually occur after you strain your voice. Shouting, long periods of singing, or simply cheering for your football team may cause you to lose your voice. In a day or two, it should return to normal.

Another form of hoarseness, commonly known as laryngitis, usually results from an acute inflammation of the mucous membranes in your larynx. This hoarseness is actually caused by swelling of your vocal cords. A viral or bacterial infection either alone or associated with a cold or flu is the usual culprit, and pain, fever, and cough are often also present.

When your hoarseness persists and is not related to straining your voice or to laryngitis, you should suspect a more serious problem. Prolonged hoarseness or a sudden change in your voice suggests a possible growth on your vocal cords. Benign nodules or polyps occur frequently in singers and in heavy smokers.

WHEN TO BE CONCERNED

Any hoarseness that resolves within a week, especially if you have strained your voice or had a recent upper respiratory infection, should not be a cause for concern. If you notice that your hoarseness comes and goes, arrange a medical evaluation, especially if you're a smoker. Any persistent hoarseness likewise requires a thorough evaluation.

TREATMENT

Treatment for hoarseness due to laryngitis basically consists of resting your voice, avoiding smoking, and controlling postnasal drainage from allergies or sinus infections. Home treatment consists of warm saltwater gargles, local hot packs on the neck, and steam inhalation. If your laryngitis is associated with a fever and is due to a bacterial infection, antibiotic medications may be indicated. If swelling is significant and risks blocking your airway, steroid medications may be necessary to reduce it.

CALL YOUR DOCTOR WHEN:

• you have hoarseness that comes and goes or that persists for longer than a week.

TOOTHACHE

DESCRIPTION

Toothache is a symptom that is characteristic of many different dental problems. Your pain will typically be a steady, gnawing ache, often with an associated swelling of your face. Most toothaches are caused by an infection of the root of the tooth. When this infection involves the soft pulp that surrounds the nerve, the tooth becomes extremely sensitive to hot or cold foods or liquids. There is also pain when the tooth is simply tapped with your finger. Other causes of toothache include impaction of a wisdom tooth or an abscess at the root of the tooth.

WHEN TO BE CONCERNED

Generally, any toothache deserves prompt dental attention. If your pain stems from an infection of the root of your tooth, early treatment may prevent it from spreading to the soft pulp surrounding the nerve. A tooth abscess is generally considered to be a dental emergency. Failure to treat an abscess promptly may result in the spread of this infection through your bloodstream. Likewise, see your dentist as soon as possible if you have an impacted molar that is causing significant pain.

TREATMENT

When the root of your tooth is infected, most commonly from bacteria in your saliva, your dentist will apply medication to try to prevent its spread to the pulp. If your infection is far advanced, he may recommend root canal surgery to remove the pulp and then sterilize and fill the canal. When you have a dental abscess, your tooth will probably need to be opened and drained. A flap of your gum may need to be cut to remove the abscess and try to save the tooth. Antibiotics will be prescribed to prevent the infection from spreading through your bloodstream.

An impacted wisdom tooth will usually be seen clearly on X-rays. Often the surrounding gum will become swollen and tender. Your dentist will try to avoid pulling the tooth if at all possible.

CALL YOUR DENTIST WHEN:

• you have a toothache.

JAW PAIN

DESCRIPTION

Your upper and lower jaw on each side of your mouth are connected by a sliding type of hinge. When this hinge is misaligned from any deviation or dislocation of your jaw, jaw pain may result. This symptom, often known as the TMJ (temporomandibular joint) syndrome, may be caused by a natural overbite, poorly fitting dentures, grinding your teeth in your sleep (bruxism), or various types of arthritis of the joint itself.

While this condition is usually not serious, it may be uncomfortable and prevent you from fully opening your mouth. Your face may become sore, and you may have difficulty in chewing and swallowing. You may hear a clicking sound when you open and close your mouth, or you may feel a grinding when you put your finger over the joint.

WHEN TO BE CONCERNED

This symptom should generally not cause alarm. The underlying cause needs to be determined, and attempts should be made to correct it. If this symptom follows an acute trauma to the joint, your doctor may request X-rays to determine if there has been an acute injury to the bone.

TREATMENT

The treatment of this symptom involves determining and treating the underlying cause. Often the condition is chronic, and your doctor will request X-rays of the joint to make the diagnosis. The acute symptoms are usually treated by keeping the jaw as immobilized as possible. Try to maintain a soft diet and avoid eating hard foods or chewing gum. You may also try tranquilizers or painkillers if your symptoms are persistent.

CALL YOUR DOCTOR WHEN:

- you have pain in your jaw associated with opening and closing your mouth.

Chapter 10

Symptoms and Diseases of the Heart and Respiratory System

CHEST PAIN

DESCRIPTION

Although many people immediately associate chest pain with a heart condition, this symptom can also result from many other far less serious problems. For example, you may experience mild chest discomfort after eating an especially heavy or spicy meal. Such simple indigestion (*see* Heartburn/Indigestion) may be alarming but is rarely serious.

Also, your chest wall contains many small muscles, ligaments, and cartilages that support your rib cage. Sometimes these structures may be strained by exercise or affected by a virus infection (pleurodynia) causing chest pain and soreness.

Another more serious cause of chest pain is a condition known as pleurisy. This symptom usually results from inflammation and scarring of the lining of the lung, which sometimes follows pneumonia or another serious lung infection. In some cases, a blood clot that has traveled to the lung or even a tumor can also cause this type of pain. The pain itself is known as pleuritic pain, and it is almost always related to your breathing. It usually becomes worse while you are taking a deep breath.

Almost everyone knows that unexplained chest pain is a symptom that should be taken seriously, especially by those at high risk of heart disease (*see* Coronary Risk Factors). Your coronary arteries normally carry an adequate amount of oxygen-filled blood to nourish your heart muscle (myocardium). Chest pain, called angina pectoris, is usually a warning signal, short of an actual heart attack, that your heart is not getting the oxygen that it needs. This pain, best described as a heaviness or pressure beneath your breastbone (sternum), usually comes on during or immediately following exertion and is relieved by rest.

You may or may not be fortunate enough to get such a warning signal of coronary artery disease. Any activity that increases your heart rate causes it to demand more oxygen. A hardening or blockage in these arteries supplying blood to your heart usually causes angina or an actual heart attack. Anything that narrows these arteries, such as a high blood cholesterol level or smoking, will increase your risk of heart disease.

Likewise, if your arteries are already narrowed by this condition, anything that further compromises this blood supply can cause an actual heart attack. Overexertion, excess caffeine, and even stress can also cause these arteries to constrict. High blood pressure and obesity further aggravate a decreased blood flow by forcing your heart to work even harder.

WHEN TO BE CONCERNED

If you are young and healthy and develop mild chest discomfort after eating a heavy or spicy meal, your symptoms are likely due to indigestion. If your symptoms are due to heartburn, they should be relieved promptly with antacids. Also, with heartburn, you should *not* experience any associated shortness of breath, increased pain on deep breathing, or movement of the pain to your jaw or arm.

Chest pain resulting from a muscle strain or an inflammation of a cartilage usually comes on gradually and follows a particularly strenuous activity such as doing push-ups. Chest pains may result from a flulike virus. Again, this type of pain is rarely associated with shortness of breath and seldom moves from your chest. If you develop this type of pain, you should still seek prompt medical attention to be certain that there is not a more serious underlying cause.

If you develop a sharp pain in your chest following a severe respiratory infection or pneumonia, particularly when you inhale deeply, suspect that you have pleuritic-type pain. This type of chest pain requires prompt medical evaluation. When your pain has come on more suddenly without an associated cough, fever, or other symptoms of a lung infection, be concerned that it may be due to a blood clot that has traveled to your lung. This is especially true if you are at high risk of developing this condition (*see* Leg Pain and Symptoms). Always consider any sudden chest pain associated with shortness of breath to be an emergency requiring *immediate* medical attention.

If you are over 30 and at high risk for a heart attack, assume that severe chest pain is due to coronary artery disease. A heart attack is especially likely if you already have a history of angina pectoris. Also, if your pain follows exertion; travels to your neck, arm, or jaw; or is associated with shortness of breath and sweating, suspect a heart attack. Anyone at high risk should be prepared for such an emergency (*see* Cardiac Arrest). Be sure your family members have taken an approved cardiopulmonary resuscitation (CPR) training course. Keep copies of recent medical records handy and know the names and locations of nearby paramedic and emergency facilities. Call for help immediately. If paramedics are not available quickly, have someone take you to the nearest emergency room. Your survival may depend on how quickly you get medical help.

TREATMENT

If you suspect that your chest discomfort is due to indigestion and you are not at high risk for heart disease or a blood clot, you may try a brief course of home treatment consisting basically of antacids. If your pain persists or occurs repeatedly, see your doctor to rule out other diseases of the digestive system.

Chest pain caused by a muscle strain or a viral inflammation is usually treated with heat, rest, and painkillers, if necessary. Pleuritic pain usually indicates a serious underlying cause. Treatment is aimed at pain relief followed by diagnosis and treatment of the underlying cause.

The treatment for angina pectoris involves a combination of reduction or elimination of cardiac risk factors, medication, and, in severe cases, when indicated, surgery. Your doctor will first confirm his suspicions with an exercise stress test. Certain characteristic changes in your EKG during exercise may indicate that your heart is not getting enough oxygen. If this test suggests a significant blockage of your coronary arteries, your doctor may suggest a cardiac catheterization. In this procedure, a dye is injected into your bloodstream to outline the blood flow through your coronary arteries.

If this test indicates only mild to moderate blockage of your coronary arteries, medical treatment will generally be tried first. Try to reduce or eliminate every risk factor. If your cholesterol is elevated, your doctor will recommend a diet and/or medication to reduce it. High blood pressure will be treated vigorously and a low-salt diet prescribed. Learn to check your blood pressure regularly at home. Stop smoking immediately! If you're overweight, this is the time to reduce. It may be your last chance. Finally, if you've been sedentary most of your life, now is the time to begin a carefully supervised exercise program.

Medical treatment for angina consists of nitroglycerin in various forms as well as a number of newer drugs. If there is a significant obstruction that appears to be surgically correctable, a bypass procedure may be indicated. Recently, certain localized types of obstruction have been corrected with a much simpler surgical procedure called balloon angioplasty.

CALL YOUR DOCTOR WHEN:

- you have severe indigestion or other digestive symptoms that regularly cause chest pain or discomfort.
- you have chest pain for any reason. *It is especially urgent that you seek immediate emergency medical care if you are at high risk for heart disease or if your chest pain is associated with shortness of breath, sweating, or pain that travels to your neck, jaw, or left arm.*

CORONARY RISK FACTORS

Correctable

Smoking

Obesity

Stressful lifestyle

High blood pressure

High cholesterol and triglycerides

Decreased lung capacity

Metabolic diseases such as diabetes or an underactive thyroid gland

Insufficient exercise

Environmental stress

Not Correctable

Family history of heart disease

Advancing age

SHORTNESS OF BREATH

DESCRIPTION

What does *shortness of breath* really mean? When you think about it, this is a confusing symptom. The greatest athletes in the world literally gasp for air after a big race or other strenuous event. Shortness of breath (*see* Cough and/or Shortness of Breath) is really the inability to get enough oxygen into your system to meet its needs. While this symptom is normal in athletes pushing themselves to the limits, it can also indicate a serious underlying condition such as asthma, emphysema, or heart failure.

Anything that decreases the amount of oxygen that your blood carries to your tissues will cause you to feel short of breath. This may occur gradually with emphysema or suddenly with an acute asthma attack. In younger people, asthma may occur from a particular allergy, while in older people it may be from environmental causes such as infection.

During an asthmatic attack, the small airways in your lungs (bronchioles) become narrowed and mucus blocks the outflow of stale air, causing you to wheeze. You may feel chest tightness but rarely actual pain. You may panic as you gasp for air, but as your symptoms clear, you'll begin coughing up the thick mucus that blocked your airways.

Emphysema is an extremely serious disease that may result from years of heavy cigarette smoking (*see* Positive Health Care, Part I). Unfortunately, if you fit this pattern, you've probably already damaged the lining of your airways. If you regularly cough up phlegm, especially when awakening, you probably have chronic bronchitis, which often leads to emphysema. Again, shortness of breath is the main symptom of this condition. But, with emphysema, your breathlessness usually comes on over a period of years. Mucus from chronic irritation clogs your airways, making it harder for your body to get the oxygen it needs.

Besides lung conditions, many heart ailments also cause shortness of breath. Normally, oxygen enters your lungs and is transferred to your blood. Your heart pumps this oxygen-rich blood to your tissues. If your heart becomes weakened and fails to pump enough blood, not enough oxygen will get to your tissues. This weakened condition is called *congestive heart failure* and may be caused by such things as high blood pressure, coronary artery disease (*see* Chest Pain), or problems with the heart valves themselves. Besides shortness of breath, other associated symptoms may include cough, fatigue, and swollen feet and ankles.

WHEN TO BE CONCERNED

If you have asthma, you're familiar with the symptoms of an attack. Otherwise, any sudden shortness of breath with wheezing should certainly alarm you. Sometimes an acute allergic reaction (*see* Generalized Itching), with hives, shortness of breath, and wheezing, may mimic a simple asthmatic attack but may be life-threatening. In fact, a severe asthma attack can last for days (status asthmaticus) and may rarely cause death.

If you're a heavy smoker, be concerned about complications from your habit. Chronic cough, chest pain, or gradually worsening shortness of breath requires *immediate* medical attention. Be honest. Tell your doctor how much you smoke because you are at higher risk of developing other diseases such as high blood pressure and heart disease.

Generally, whenever you notice any shortness of breath, you should seek *immediate* medical attention. When this symptom is complicated by other symptoms of heart failure, you'll require prolonged and specialized care. Often these symptoms develop gradually, and it may be a while before you notice increasing fatigue, shortness of breath, swollen ankles, and a steady weight gain as you retain fluid. Existing high blood pressure, obesity, or a known heart condition suggests congestive heart failure until proven otherwise.

TREATMENT

Home treatment for asthma consists of eliminating the cause, if possible; taking prescribed medications; and drinking lots of fluids. More severe cases may require a trip to an emergency room for a shot of adrenaline or one of the new and more potent drugs now available to control difficult cases. Often, when the cause can be identified, a program of desensitization will be effective.

Obviously, the most effective home treatment for any symptom caused by smoking is simply to *stop smoking!* Once you are noticeably short of breath or develop other symptoms requiring medical care, you've likely suffered irreparable lung damage. While you can't undo this damage, stopping immediately will usually prevent further destruction of your lungs. At home, use air filters to prevent further lung irritation from dust. Steam inhalation may ease your breathing, and drinking lots of fluids will help to thin the mucus. Medical treatment for emphysema consists of drugs to loosen the mucus blocking your airways, drugs to expand your air passages, and antibiotics to treat infection.

Treating congestive heart failure involves diagnosis and treatment of the underlying cause. You'll need to lose weight, maintain a low-salt diet, and carefully take your prescribed medications. In general, once your doctor completely evaluates your condition, the mainstays of your medical management will be diuretics and Digitalis as well as other appropriate medications.

CALL YOUR DOCTOR WHEN:

- you are an asthmatic and develop shortness of breath that you can't control quickly with home treatment.
- you suddenly develop shortness of breath unrelated to vigorous exercise.
- you notice a shortness of breath that has begun gradually and gotten worse over a period of time.

COUGH

DESCRIPTION

Coughing can be a natural way for your body to remove minor irritants from your airways, or it can be a symptom of an underlying illness such as a cold or flu, bronchitis, or pneumonia (*see* Cough and/or Shortness of Breath).

The common cold (*see* Cold) usually begins with symptoms of nasal congestion and drainage (*see* Postnasal Drip). At least 40 different viruses cause common cold symptoms, and several more strains produce flulike illnesses. Both cold and flu viruses irritate the lining of your airways and produce a cough. Normally, with a simple cold, you won't run a fever of over 100 degrees Fahrenheit, even with a cough. With a flulike syndrome, you may have a higher temperature, weakness, and muscle aches and pains. Your cough with either a cold or flu will usually be dry, and you'll rarely experience shortness of breath or significant chest pain.

A cough due to bronchitis is more serious. Bronchitis is an inflammation of the lining of your airways that usually produces more mucus than a cough from a cold. This mucus blocks your air flow and must be coughed up. When the irritation causing your cough is short-lived, it is called acute bronchitis, but when it persists for several months, as in heavy cigarette smokers, it is termed chronic bronchitis.

Acute bronchitis is often a bacterial complication of a cold, flu, or other respiratory infection. With this, expect a temperature as high as 102 and a cough producing thick, yellowish sputum. With chronic bronchitis, especially resulting from heavy cigarette smoking, your cough will be constant and usually worse on awakening. Chronic bronchitis is often linked to emphysema (*see* Shortness of Breath). With this you may run a low-grade fever. Your chronically weakened condition may make you more susceptible to bouts of acute bronchitis or pneumonia.

While bronchitis is often a chronic irritation of your airways that produces a cough, pneumonia is an acute inflammation of the air sacs in your lungs themselves. Besides bacteria, viruses and even fungi can also cause these air sacs to fill with pus and fluid. A virus usually causes milder symptoms than a bacterial pneumonia, but both are marked by coughing, fatigue, chest congestion, and fever.

With a bacterial pneumonia, your fever may be as high as 104 degrees Fahrenheit, and your cough will produce a thick, dark, yellowish or rust-colored sputum. You may also have shaking chills and shortness of breath in severe cases.

WHEN TO BE CONCERNED

The main danger of a cold or flu is that it lowers your resistance. In children, the elderly, or those with a chronic debilitating illness such as diabetes or heart disease, be concerned about a more serious complication. Bacteria, normally in your system, can cause pneumonia, bronchitis, sinusitis, or other infections.

When your cough is persistent and produces a thick yellowish mucus, suspect bronchitis. A low-grade fever, chest congestion, wheezing, and possibly shortness of breath are also clues to acute bronchitis. As the condition worsens, your cough becomes heavier and the mucus becomes thicker. Once you are wheezing and short of breath, your condition is serious. If acute bronchitis is not treated promptly, chronic bronchitis or other complications may develop.

The sudden onset of high fever; chills; a severe cough producing a thick, yellowish sputum; chest congestion; and shortness of breath requires *immediate* medical attention. While pneumonia commonly occurs in already weak and debilitated people, it may also occur if you are otherwise healthy.

TREATMENT

For a mild cough due to a cold or flu, home treatment should include rest, increased fluids, steam inhalation, and possibly an expectorant. Cold and flu are viral diseases and are not affected by antibiotics. In fact, repeated, unnecessary use of antibiotics can be harmful. Most cough suppressants will only mask your symptoms and dry your air passages. Some experts believe they may actually prolong your cough. Expectorants, on the other hand, provide relief by breaking up the congestion, enabling you to cough up the mucus.

Treating bronchitis involves clearing the mucus from your air passages, removing irritants, and treating the infection. If your bronchitis stems from smoking, stop immediately! Steam inhalation may help to loosen mucus. Drink lots of fluids and try to cough up the mucus. Your doctor may prescribe antibiotics to fight infection and also drugs called bronchodilators to help open your airways. If you have chronic bronchitis or another debilitating illness, your doctor may recommend vaccination for flu and pneumonia.

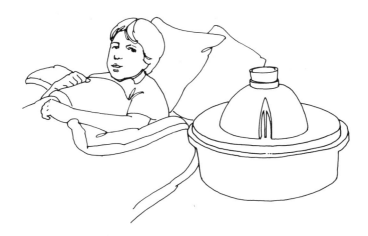

CALL YOUR DOCTOR WHEN:

- you have any cough that persists for more than a week.
- you have a cold or flu with a cough and a fever of over 102 degrees Fahrenheit.
- you have the sudden onset of a cough with fever and chills.

ABNORMAL HEARTBEAT

DESCRIPTION

Your heart should normally beat at regular intervals to pump a steady supply of blood through your body. Although everyone has a fairly slow resting pulse, each person's will be different, depending on their level of physical conditioning as well as other factors such as basic metabolism. Similarly, vigorous exercise (*see* Physical Fitness) as well as other activities or emotions such as fear and anger will normally increase everyone's heart rate. An abnormal heartbeat is usually caused by an abnormally slow or fast heartbeat or by an irregular heart rhythm.

If you regularly engage in vigorous exercise, your resting heart rate may be as low as 50 beats per minute. Most athletes have a slow heart rate, and experts believe this is healthy since it places less stress on the heart. However, a slow heart rate that is not simply due to good conditioning can be a symptom of a serious underlying disorder.

For example, if the conduction system of your heart is blocked, you can have an abnormally slow pulse. Also, if you're recovering from a prolonged illness following weeks of bed rest, your pulse may be slow. Although most illnesses, particularly infections, elevate your heart rate, some infections may actually do the opposite. Certain types of poisoning as well as an underactive thyroid gland may also cause a slow pulse. Since your brain is the organ most sensitive to a decreased blood supply, an abnormally slowed heart rate is often associated with dizziness and fainting.

A rapid heartbeat can simply be your body's normal response to vigorous exercise or to fear or anger. Likewise, various illnesses such as infections, an overactive thyroid gland, anemia, and lung disease will also increase your heart rate. Also, many drugs, as well as caffeine, alcohol, and tobacco, will have the same effect. A rapid heartbeat is also seen in pregnancy, obesity, menopause, and various gastrointestinal diseases. In older folks, a persistently rapid heartbeat is often a symptom of heart disease. The symptoms of a rapid heartbeat are usually shortness of breath, fever, cough, or chest pain.

While everyone's heart "skips a beat" occasionally, frequent or serious irregularities in your heartbeat can cause grave problems such as dizziness, fainting, chest pain, or even a heart attack. Most "palpitations" are caused by foods, drugs, or emotional upset rather than by a serious underlying disease. Drugs such as atropine, belladonna, and adrenaline, as well as other substances such as coffee, alcohol, tea, and a multitude of food additives, often cause an irregular heartbeat, which also may result from emotional upset or from overexertion.

Sometimes an irregular heartbeat is a symptom of a serious underlying illness. Your heart is controlled partly by a small area of nerve tissue (sinoatrial node) in the heart itself. Any injury to this conduction system from infection, drugs, or even a prior heart attack can cause an irregular heartbeat. Besides abnormalities in the heart, many other conditions, such as lung disease, anemia, and hormonal imbalances like those found in menopause or with an overactive thyroid gland, may make your heart beat irregularly.

WHEN TO BE CONCERNED

If you're very athletic and have a resting pulse rate near 50 without any symptoms, don't be concerned. But, if you are basically sedentary and notice a very slow pulse, have your doctor check to be sure there is no underlying cause such as an underactive thyroid gland. Regardless of your activity, if your pulse is slow and you experience light-headedness or fainting, see your doctor *immediately*.

If you rarely exercise and your resting pulse is usually over 80, arrange a routine medical exam and begin a supervised exercise program. A resting pulse that is over 100 for more than an hour or two and is unrelated to food, alcohol, drugs, a fever, or an emotional upset requires prompt medical evaluation to determine the cause. When other symptoms such as chest pain, dizziness, or fainting are associated with a rapid heartbeat, *immediate* medical care is required.

Most palpitations caused by certain foods or drugs generally shouldn't worry you as long as they go away. Otherwise, irregular heartbeats that occur more than just occasionally or persist for more than a few minutes deserve a careful medical evaluation. Palpitations that occur when you exercise should cause concern because they should stop when your heart rate increases. If you are at high risk for heart disease or have had a previous heart attack, any heart irregularity requires *immediate* medical care. Likewise, if your palpitations are associated with other symptoms such as chest pain, dizziness, or fainting, see your doctor *immediately*.

TREATMENT

There is basically no home treatment for any abnormality of your heartbeat except avoiding stress and irritating substances. Medical treatment for these abnormalities first requires a careful medical history and a complete examination to determine the underlying problem, including an EKG as well as other more sophisticated tests.

If a cause of your abnormality can be found, it will be treated. If the problem involves your heart itself, this will need careful evaluation. In many cases, no underlying cause will be found for an abnormal heartbeat. Depending on your particular case, your doctor may recommend one of many new drugs available along with regular medical follow-up care. Severe cases that can't be controlled with medication alone may require pacemakers or other surgical techniques.

CALL YOUR DOCTOR WHEN:

- you do not exercise vigorously and you notice a slow heart rate near 50 or you experience dizziness or fainting.
- you notice a rapid heartbeat that does not go away when you avoid certain substances or you experience a rapid heartbeat associated with fever, shortness of breath, or other symptoms (*call immediately*).
- you experience palpitations that occur repeatedly, that persist for more than a few minutes, or that are associated with any other symptoms.

HEART MURMURS

DESCRIPTION

Your heart contains four chambers along with four valves that control the flow of blood between the chambers. As these valves open and close, they normally make sounds that you can hear when you put your ear to someone's chest. Many heart murmurs are found during routine physical exams. With a stethoscope, your doctor can easily hear these sounds.

One or more of these valves may be abnormal at birth or may be damaged as a result of infection, injury, or calcification. This causes changes in the normal sounds that the blood makes as it rushes through your heart. Other conditions also can change the usual sounds your heart makes. These different sounds are often called heart murmurs.

WHEN TO BE CONCERNED

There are many types of heart murmurs, and not all are due to serious heart disease. Sometimes heart murmurs come and go, especially in children. They may occur only when you are in a certain position or only during an acute illness. Many people live out their entire lives normally despite loud murmurs that may have been present since childhood. Although a murmur, in many cases, will not be associated with other medical problems, any heart murmur deserves a thorough medical evaluation.

If your heart murmur is related to other heart symptoms such as chest pain (*see* Chest Pain), shortness of breath (*see* Shortness of Breath), dizziness (*see* Dizziness), or fainting (*see* Loss of Consciousness), *immediate* medical attention is required. Almost all serious murmurs are associated with other more obvious symptoms.

TREATMENT

Obviously, there is no home treatment for a heart murmur. If you have a murmur, your doctor must determine its cause. A great many sophisticated tests are now available to analyze and evaluate the function of your heart. Aside from a routine EKG, your doctor may request ultrasound studies of your heart valves. In serious cases, where other symptoms are present, more involved studies may be necessary, and you may even require surgery to correct a serious defect.

CALL YOUR DOCTOR WHEN:

• you first become aware that you have a heart murmur.

Chapter 11

Symptoms and Diseases of the Digestive System

HEARTBURN/INDIGESTION

DESCRIPTION

Heartburn, indigestion, and bloating are perhaps the most common digestive symptoms that people experience. Your esophagus is a muscular tube that connects your throat with your stomach. Since this tube passes behind your breastbone alongside your heart, any irritation or inflammation here is commonly known as "heartburn." This symptom is usually described as a burning in the chest, often accompanied by difficulty in swallowing. This inflammation of the lining can be either acute or chronic.

If you experience a burning pain behind your breastbone that begins soon after a spicy meal, excessive vomiting, or heavy smoking, you may well have an acute inflammation of the esophagus. Your pain will usually come on slowly an hour or so after meals. Because your esophagus is so close to your heart, lungs, and stomach, pain originating here may sometimes mimic a more serious condition in these other organs.

Sometimes a small pocket (hiatal hernia) may develop near your diaphragm where your esophagus connects to your stomach. This condition is fairly common, especially in obese people. In some cases, when this occurs, the normal digestive acids from your stomach spill into this pocket, causing a chronic inflammation. This is known as reflux esophagitis and is often a chronic condition. Most people with a hiatal hernia don't even know they have it, but others frequently suffer from symptoms of heartburn described above.

Indigestion is really a group of symptoms that includes gas and bloating as well as heartburn. Bloating is usually caused by an abnormal amount of air in your stomach or intestines. This symptom usually results from swallowing large amounts of air when you eat quickly and gulp your food. Also, nervous and tense people as well as many gum chewers and smokers tend to swallow air. Finally, certain foods such as bran, cabbage, beer, and carbonated beverages are notorious causes of gas.

WHEN TO BE CONCERNED

Heartburn usually comes on slowly an hour or so after a particularly heavy or spicy meal. You'll usually describe your pain as a burning feeling beneath your breastbone that lasts for a few hours. If this is merely caused by a mild irritation of your esophagus, don't be overly concerned. Many people mistake heartburn and indigestion for symptoms of a heart attack. Heartburn and indigestion are rarely associated with sweating or shortness of breath. Also, pain from heartburn rarely travels to your neck, jaw, or left arm.

If you frequently have symptoms of heartburn, regardless of what you eat, and you seem to get little relief from antacids, you may have a hiatal hernia with chronic esophagitis. See your doctor as soon as possible. On the other hand, a burning pain in your stomach that improves when you eat suggests a possible ulcer (*see* Abdominal Cramping and Distention) and requires prompt medical attention. Symptoms of weight loss, severe abdominal pain, or gastrointestinal bleeding (bloody vomitus or stools) require *immediate* medical attention.

If you suffer from frequent indigestion with bloating and gas despite a change in your habits, arrange for a medical evaluation. These symptoms may be a clue to other digestive problems, perhaps involving your gallbladder or pancreas. Sudden weight loss (*see* Weight Loss or Loss of Appetite) with or without a loss of appetite is a serious digestive symptom that requires *immediate* attention.

If you are at high risk for a heart attack (*see* Chest Pain), always be concerned about any pain deep in your chest. Be sure you don't pass off a warning of heart disease as simply indigestion.

TREATMENT

Home treatment of mild esophagitis requires that you stop smoking and avoid eating hot or spicy foods and lie down immediately after meals. Antacids should promptly relieve your symptoms.

Most people seldom have symptoms of gas and bloating. If you often feel bloated, try eating several smaller and more leisurely meals. Avoid drinking large amounts of water or carbonated beverages with meals and also try to stop chewing gum and smoking.

If your heartburn or indigestion persists, you'll need a careful medical evaluation of your precise symptoms since your treatment will depend on the underlying cause. Your doctor may request specialized X-rays as well as other studies to determine the reason for your symptoms.

CALL YOUR DOCTOR WHEN:

- you suffer from heartburn that occurs more than occasionally or is not relieved promptly by antacids.
- you frequently experience gas or bloating despite a change in your habits.
- you have a history of or are at high risk for heart disease and you experience any pain or burning beneath your breastbone.

ABDOMINAL CRAMPING AND DISTENTION

DESCRIPTION

Symptoms of abdominal cramping and distention or swelling can be caused by something as common as mild gastroenteritis (*see* Nausea and Vomiting) or as life-threatening as cancer or a sudden internal hemorrhage. Ulcers, gallstones, and pancreatitis, among other conditions, may produce many confusing symptoms. Sometimes minor problems may cause worse symptoms than more serious problems do. For example, cramping from simple constipation or gas (*see* Heartburn/Indigestion) sometimes can be more painful than a tumor.

Ulceration in your digestive tract usually occurs either in your stomach (gastric) or in the first portion of your small intestine (duodenal). Ulcers are most commonly caused by today's stressful lifestyles. This stress often causes increased acid secretion and eventually leads to a small erosion or ulcer in the lining of your stomach or duodenum. Ulcers may also be caused by various medications such as aspirin or steroids, and they often complicate certain conditions such as burns or lung disease.

For some reason, gallbladder disease is much more common in women than in men. It is often associated with obesity and occurs most commonly in middle age. Although your gallbladder may be the site of a tumor, stones in your gallbladder or bile duct most frequently cause problems. While many people have gallstones their entire lives without symptoms, others develop every symptom and complication. Once a stone causes a blockage, inflammation (cholecystitis), infection (cholangitis), and even a perforation may follow. Discomfort *after* meals; belching; flatulence; abdominal cramping, especially beneath your right breast; and sometimes a yellowish cast to your skin (jaundice) (*see* Skin Discolorations) all strongly suggest gallbladder disease.

Your pancreas is a large gland lying behind your stomach. Like your gallbladder, it normally secretes digestive enzymes. Inflammation of the pancreas usually occurs in people who have gallbladder disease or in heavy drinkers. Sometimes infections elsewhere, such as mumps, hepatitis, or mononucleosis, have been known to lead to pancreatitis.

WHEN TO BE CONCERNED

The most common symptom of an ulcer is a burning ache between your navel and breastbone that occurs often, especially when your stomach is empty. Your pain may be relieved temporarily by antacids, by vomiting, or simply by eating. Although sometimes ulcers occur at the site of a tumor, the main danger is the risk of perforation or hemorrhage. Any abdominal burning or cramping pain that persists for more than a few hours should cause concern. If there are other associated symptoms such as severe pain, a fever, bloody stools, or vomitus that may resemble coffee grounds, seek *immediate* medical attention.

Pain beneath your right breast that comes on after meals and is associated with cramping, belching, distention, and flatulence is suggestive of gallbladder disease. A yellowish cast to your skin should give you a definite clue. Any of these symptoms warrants a thorough medical evaluation.

An acute inflammation of your pancreas usually causes severe cramping pain in your upper abdomen that may travel to your back. If you're a heavy drinker or already have gallbladder disease, you are at high risk for pancreatitis. This condition may come on suddenly, and you may become quite sick, with cold clammy skin, nausea, and vomiting. Pancreatitis requires *immediate* medical care.

TREATMENT

If you have even mild symptoms that suggest an ulcer, see your doctor to confirm this diagnosis before attempting home treatment. If you have a mild ulcer, home treatment consists of following a careful diet, eating smaller and more frequent meals, and taking antacids regularly. Don't overlook changing the stressful lifestyle that probably led to your ulcer in the first place. If your symptoms don't respond promptly, other drugs to decrease the acid secretion may be necessary. Emergency surgery is almost always required for complications of bleeding or perforation.

Whenever gallbladder disease is suspected, it must be confirmed with special X-rays. If your symptoms are mild, your doctor may suggest a special diet avoiding all fried or greasy foods as well as certain gas-forming vegetables. If your symptoms are severe or persist, surgical removal of gallstones is usually recommended.

Suspect pancreatitis as the cause of severe upper abdominal pain that travels to your back. Seek *immediate* medical diagnosis and treatment. If your doctor confirms this diagnosis, he'll put you on complete bed rest and begin intravenous fluids. Your stomach will be kept completely empty through suction, and medications will be prescribed to cut down the secretions from your pancreas. Antibiotics may be used to prevent infection of your abdominal cavity.

CALL YOUR DOCTOR WHEN:

- you have burning or cramping abdominal pain that persists for more than a few hours or occurs repeatedly.
- your pain is severe or associated with fever or evidence of bleeding.
- you notice a yellowish cast to your skin.

NAUSEA AND VOMITING

DESCRIPTION

Most of us have experienced nausea and even vomiting at one time or another. Nausea can best be described as a very uncomfortable feeling in the stomach accompanied by an urge to vomit. Vomiting is the forceful and uncontrollable ejection of the stomach contents. What most people don't realize is that nausea and the urge to vomit are actually triggered from an area of the brain. This area receives information from your digestive system and, in some cases, from the nerves in your inner ear that control your sense of balance.

Most episodes of nausea are temporary, and you may or may not also experience vomiting and abdominal cramps. Occasionally, an acute episode of nausea and vomiting may even be beneficial to you. These symptoms may be your body's normal defense against the intake of a harmful substance.

Nausea and vomiting usually result from such common conditions as viral gastroenteritis, pregnancy, and motion sickness. Other common causes of nausea and vomiting are eating spoiled food, eating in excess, emotional upset, drinking excess alcohol, and side effects from medications. When you are nauseated from one of these causes, you may also experience chills, sweating, rapid heartbeat, and headache.

WHEN TO BE CONCERNED

If you are suffering from prolonged or repeated nausea with vomiting, you may risk a serious depletion of your body fluids, salts, and nutrients. Also, persistent vomiting may cause damage to the lining of your stomach and esophagus. Prolonged and repeated vomiting should lead you to seek medical attention. Your doctor will check you carefully for more serious causes of these symptoms, such as gastritis, peptic ulcers, hepatitis, or pancreatitis. If you are vomiting blood or a substance with the appearance of coffee grounds, you must seek *immediate* medical attention. Vomiting without nausea may also follow severe abdominal injury or head injuries and likewise requires *immediate* attention.

TREATMENT

You will find that both nausea and vomiting will usually subside once the cause has been corrected. The common causes of vomiting usually require no treatment other than removal of the offending substance. Vomiting during morning sickness of pregnancy also usually requires no treatment, but you should advise your obstetrician if these symptoms become severe.

While your symptoms will usually resolve in a day or two, you should stay on small amounts of a clear liquid diet for the first 12 hours (*see* Diet for the Control of Vomiting). These liquids may include tea, soft drinks, soup broth, and apple juice. It is important that you replace the fluids your body is losing and avoid becoming dehydrated. You should avoid solid food until your vomiting has stopped. At this point, you should begin by eating small pieces of crackers or toast and gradually return to your normal diet.

If your symptoms of vomiting continue for longer than one or two days, you should visit your doctor. If this becomes necessary, it will be helpful if you bring along a sample of your vomitus. At this point, your doctor will examine you thoroughly and may prescribe medication to help control your nausea and vomiting. If necessary, your doctor may order certain diagnostic laboratory and X-ray studies to evaluate your symptoms further. *It is important that you inform your doctor if you think you may be pregnant since certain medications or tests may harm your baby.*

CALL YOUR DOCTOR WHEN:

- your nausea and vomiting persist for more than two days.
- your nausea and vomiting are associated with severe abdominal pain, high fever, or bloody vomitus (*call immediately*).
- your nausea and vomiting result from the ingestion of a toxic substance.
- you suspect that you may be pregnant.
- your nausea and vomiting result from abdominal trauma or head injury.
- your vomitus contains what look like coffee grounds (*call immediately*).

DIET FOR THE CONTROL OF VOMITING

During the first 12 hours after vomiting has begun, limit yourself to clear liquids in small amounts. Avoid dairy products, citrus juice, and solid foods. Recommended liquids are:

- water
- sweet fruit juices (apple, peach, grape)
- bouillon
- flavored gelatin
- softened popsicles
- carbonated beverages (stirred to remove bubbles)

During the next 12 hours, continue frequent small amounts of the fluids listed above. Gradually add foods from the list below. Avoid dairy products—including eggs, butter, cheese, and milk—and citrus fruits and juices.

- applesauce
- banana
- toast and jelly (no butter)
- soup (not creamed)
- soda crackers
- rice
- dry sweetened cereals
- pretzels

After 24 hours, begin to add foods from the following list:

- broiled chicken (skin removed)
- lean beef
- apple (peeled)
- cottage cheese
- tapioca pudding
- boiled, cooled nonfat milk

Gradually add more foods during the next two or three days. Return to a regular diet gradually. If vomiting persists, consult your doctor.

CHANGE IN BOWEL HABITS

DESCRIPTION

Most people hardly give their bowel habits a second thought. But any persistent change in your normal pattern can be a serious symptom requiring careful medical evaluation. Your large and small intestine are basically muscular tubes with a mucous membrane lining and a rich blood supply. Many symptoms, including cramping and abdominal distention (*see* Abdominal Cramping and Distention), can arise here. However, diarrhea and constipation are the most common bowel symptoms that almost all of us experience at some time in our lives.

Alternating diarrhea and constipation lasting longer than four or five days or recurring, especially at times of emotional stress, is usually due to an "irritable colon." Other more serious conditions that may also cause these symptoms are ulcerative colitis and diverticulosis. Tumors both inside and outside the intestine may sometimes obstruct the normal passage of stool, causing constipation.

Apart from the common cold, irritable colon is probably mankind's most common malady. Like colitis, this milder condition usually occurs in anxiety-ridden people living stressful lifestyles. Such stresses as losing your job or getting a divorce may cause your symptoms to flare up. The symptoms may include diarrhea, constipation, and stools covered with mucus but without bleeding or a fever. Abdominal cramping and distention as well as vomiting and loss of appetite are other symptoms often seen.

Diverticulitis is caused by an inflammation of small pockets that sometimes form in the wall of the colon. Many people develop these pockets during middle age, but only about 20 percent of these actually develop inflammation. These infected pockets may perforate, causing a life-threatening emergency. If the infection remains mild and chronic, symptoms may include diarrhea that alternates with constipation, fever, and intermittent pain in your left lower abdomen.

Ulcerative colitis is a serious and often chronic inflammation of the mucous membrane lining your colon. Although its cause is uncertain, many experts believe stress and emotional upset are major factors. This serious and often incapacitating condition usually comes on in middle age, although it may affect younger people. Severe and often bloody diarrhea is the main symptom of ulcerative colitis with as many as a dozen bowel movements a day. Other symptoms include abdominal cramps, weight loss, loss of appetite, and a moderate fever. This is a serious medical problem requiring long-term medical management.

WHEN TO BE CONCERNED

Generally, any change in your bowel habits that lasts more than four or five days should concern you. If you're generally anxious and have undergone a recent emotional stress, suspect an irritable colon. You may experience alternating periods of diarrhea and constipation, but you should not have any bleeding, significant weight loss, or fever. Rectal bleeding (your stools may be black or tarry) from anything other than hemorrhoids (*see* Rectal Pain and Bleeding) should cause alarm and requires *immediate* medical care.

If you are middle-aged and have alternating diarrhea and constipation along with fever but without a significant weight loss or bleeding, you may well have diverticulosis. A fever and weight loss along with mucus-covered, bloody diarrhea are suspicious symptoms suggesting ulcerative colitis. Any of these three symptoms associated with abdominal pain requires *immediate* medical care.

TREATMENT

Since an irritable colon is almost always caused by emotional factors, treatment involves reassurance that irritable bowel is not a serious condition, counseling, and elimination of enemas and laxatives. A bland diet (*see* Diet to Control Diarrhea), relaxation, and lots of exercise are usually recommended. Attempt to have bowel movements at the same time each day. Relax and try to release your tensions through exercise. If your diarrhea is severe, your doctor may prescribe antispasmodics and tranquilizers.

Diverticulitis is usually diagnosed by X-ray and requires conservative management by your doctor. This will usually include a liquid diet, bed rest, and antibiotic medications. If your diarrhea is severe, antispasmodic drugs may be prescribed.

Despite the obvious severity of the symptoms, ulcerative colitis is usually confirmed by X-rays. Often your doctor will visually inspect your colon and possibly take a biopsy. Treatment of acute attacks consists of bed rest, increased fluids, and a carefully controlled diet. If the diarrhea is severe, your doctor may prescribe antispasmodics. Steroid enemas sometimes relieve the inflammation. Severe cases may require surgery.

CALL YOUR DOCTOR WHEN:

- you notice any change in your normal bowel habits that persists for more than four or five days.
- you have fever and/or rectal bleeding associated with your bowel movements.

DIET TO CONTROL DIARRHEA

Eliminate all fruits (apples or bananas, however, may not cause problems).

During the first 12 hours after diarrhea, limit yourself to clear liquids. Avoid dairy products, citrus juices, and solid foods. Recommended liquids are:

- water
- sweet fruit juices
- flavored gelatin
- bouillon

During the next 12 hours, continue fluids and gradually add foods from the list below. Continue to avoid dairy products and citrus fruits and juices.

- applesauce
- banana
- soup
- rice
- dry cereals
- toast
- crackers

Gradually return to a regular diet.

RECTAL PAIN AND BLEEDING

DESCRIPTION

Rectal pain and bleeding are perhaps two of the most embarrassing and bothersome symptoms that you may ever encounter. Although most conditions causing these symptoms are not life-threatening, delays in diagnosis and treatment may lead to serious long-term problems.

Hemorrhoids, or "piles," as they are often called, are easily the most common cause of rectal pain and bleeding. These small, swollen, and painful clusters of veins just inside or outside your rectum can be caused by any number of things. They are common in pregnancy, in the obese, and in constipation with straining during bowel movements. If your hemorrhoids protrude from your rectum, you may first notice itching. As they become more irritated and swollen from bowel movements, they may become more painful and begin to bleed. Sometimes the blood in these swollen veins may clot (thrombose), and the veins may ulcerate.

The mucous membranes that line the rectum also contain glands that may become infected and form pockets of pus. If not treated promptly by your doctor, these infections can spread to the deep tissues around your rectum and become quite painful, especially during a bowel movement. Once a rectal abscess develops, you'll experience symptoms of fever and rectal spasm.

Your rectum is actually the last several inches of your colon. Any inflammatory condition of the colon (colitis) (*see* Change in Bowel Habits) can extend into the rectum. Likewise, your rectum can become inflamed from laxatives, hard stools, drugs, or allergies. Any such inflammation of this area is known as proctitis. The main symptom of this condition is spasm and difficulty passing stool.

WHEN TO BE CONCERNED

If you have significant rectal bleeding or pain, you should seek *immediate* medical care. Scanty rectal bleeding or pain (even when you can see the problem) still requires a careful medical evaluation. Do not assume that all rectal bleeding is simply due to hemorrhoids.

Rectal pain, especially when associated with fever, needs prompt evaluation. These may be symptoms of a rectal abscess or proctitis.

TREATMENT

Once your doctor has determined that hemorrhoids are the only reason for your rectal symptoms, he'll try to correct any underlying cause. At home, watch your diet and avoid irritating and constipating foods. Take regular hot sitz baths and use laxatives and local medications when necessary. If your symptoms are severe and not relieved by home treatment, routine surgery may provide relief.

Generally, there is no effective home treatment once a rectal abscess has developed. Antibiotics alone, without surgical drainage, are usually not very effective. Once this condition has been diagnosed and treated surgically, your doctor may recommend a special diet, sitz baths, and antibiotics. Early surgical drainage usually prevents long-term complications.

Treatment of proctitis basically involves identification and treatment of the underlying problem. Your doctor may prescribe medication to relieve the pain and spasm. He may also recommend suppositories, sitz baths, and hot packs to help relieve your symptoms.

CALL YOUR DOCTOR WHEN:

- you have rectal pain or bleeding, regardless of the cause.

Chapter 12

Symptoms and Diseases of the Urinary Tract

FREQUENT URINATION

DESCRIPTION

If you are like most people, you urinate about four to six times a day. If you are urinating more frequently and not taking fluid pills or drinking more fluids, this could be a symptom of a bladder infection. If you are taking in more fluids because you've just decided to increase your intake, frequent urination is normal. However, if you are drinking more because you've become thirstier lately, especially if you have associated blurred vision, fatigue, and weight loss despite a normal or increased appetite, see your doctor *immediately*. These could be symptoms of diabetes.

Bladder inflammation (cystitis), a relatively common urinary tract infection (especially in women), produces mild stretching of the bladder. This causes pain and urgency to urinate as well as frequent urination and occasionally blood in the urine. Typically, the amount of urine is small and the desire to urinate almost constant until the infection is treated. If you gradually develop cystitis, your first symptom will usually be frequent urination, especially at night.

Cystitis is generally caused by bacteria. Numerous bacteria normally around the urinary opening (urethra) in women may be pushed inside the urethra and/or the bladder during intercourse, causing infection. Other organisms may be introduced from the vagina, the rectum, or outside sources, including fingers and foreign objects.

In men over 50, enlargement of the prostate gland may impede flow of urine out of the bladder, causing urine to collect. This may promote the growth of bacteria and lead to infection.

WHEN TO BE CONCERNED

If you have been drinking more fluids, expect to urinate more frequently. Also, if you are taking fluid pills (diuretics) or drinking coffee or tea, which act like diuretics, you will urinate more. However, if your increased urination is associated with other symptoms described earlier, consult your physician.

TREATMENT

Treatment of frequent urination depends on why you have it. If your doctor determines that you have a bladder infection, he will treat you with antibiotics. Take all the medication prescribed to ensure a complete cure. Although cystitis usually is not a serious problem, if it is not treated promptly and completely, it may lead to a chronic infection that can persist with periodic flare-ups for months and even years. Drink plenty of fluids with your medication and urinate frequently.

Women can prevent cystitis by urinating frequently, especially just before and just after intercourse; by observing good hygiene practices to prevent unnecessary contamination from the rectum or soiled underwear; by avoiding local irritants such as bubble bath, perfumed douches, feminine hygiene sprays, and deodorant tampons. Both men and women should avoid intimate contact with anyone who has a sexually transmissible disease.

CALL YOUR DOCTOR WHEN:

- you have frequent urination without an increased fluid intake.
- you have frequent urination with an increased fluid intake and associated symptoms of fatigue, increased thirst, weight loss, and/or blurred vision.

BURNING ON URINATION

DESCRIPTION

If you experience a burning sensation when you urinate, something's wrong. Painful urination suggests irritation or inflammation, often from an infection in the urinary bladder (cystitis) or urethra (urethritis) or, in men, the prostate gland (prostatitis).

Cystitis can occur at any age and in either sex, but it is most common in women. This is because the opening to the urethra in females is close to both the rectum and the vagina, where bacteria and other organisms are normally found. When these organisms find their way into the urethra, they may move up to the bladder, causing infection.

Cystitis in men over 50 typically results from an enlarged prostate gland's blocking the flow of urine out of the bladder. As bacteria in the urine multiply, they cause inflammation and swelling of the bladder lining, which produces painful urination. This is often associated with an urge to urinate and frequent urination (see Frequent Urination). Bloody urine may also occur with cystitis (see Blood in the Urine).

The urethra is the tube that carries urine from your bladder to the outside of your body. In both men and women, glands lining this tube may harbor any bacterium or virus that gains access to the urethra. Until recently, gonorrhea was the most common cause of urethritis in young men. Today the number one cause is an organism known as chlamydia. Both infections are transmitted from one sexual partner to another. Besides painful urination, there may be itching of the urethral opening with a discharge that may be thick and greenish-yellow, indicating probable gonorrhea, or thin and watery-white, suggestive of chlamydia.

In men, bacteria may reach the prostate gland from the bloodstream or from the urethra. That's why prostatitis is commonly associated with urethritis. If the infection is acute, the first symptom may be burning on urination, usually associated with discharge from the urethra, frequent urination, fever, and groin pain. If the infection becomes chronic, there may be back pain as well.

WHEN TO BE CONCERNED

Because painful urination suggests infection, you should always consult your doctor if you experience this symptom. Untreated, infections of the urinary tract can lead to serious complications.

TREATMENT

Whenever you complain of burning on urination, your doctor will want to examine a sample of your urine under a microscope to determine if bacteria are present. If there is an infection, he'll probably prescribe antibiotics. Generally, 7–10 days of therapy will bring cystitis, urethritis, or prostatitis under control. If the diagnosis is either gonorrhea or chlamydia, any sexual partners should be treated at the same time. Women may have associated vaginal infections for which appropriate medication will be given (*see* Vaginal Discharge and Itching).

If the burning persists, and no infection is found, your doctor will carefully evaluate your bladder and urethra. He may request studies, including X-rays.

CALL YOUR DOCTOR WHEN:

• you notice burning on urination.

BLOOD IN THE URINE

DESCRIPTION

If you notice that your urine has turned red, don't panic. First, red urine doesn't always mean that blood is present. Certain foods like beets and rhubarb or drugs like Pyridium may also discolor your urine. Second, if blood is present, it may not be serious.

Blood may appear temporarily after strenuous exercise such as jogging, after a blunt injury to the back (as in football), or with a fever. Although you should notify your doctor when you have this symptom, he may only need to do a simple urinalysis.

If the blood in your urine is associated with severe back or flank pain, you may be trying to pass a kidney stone. If you have pain with urination as well as frequent and urgent urination, you may have a bladder infection (*see* Frequent Urination).

WHEN TO BE CONCERNED

If your urine looks red and you have been eating foods like beets or rhubarb, stop eating these and see if the color goes away. If so, don't worry. Also, if you're taking a medication that your doctor has warned may discolor your urine, relax. In other cases, red urine means blood is present until proven otherwise. Although blood in the urine may not be serious, always consult your physician promptly when you experience this symptom.

TREATMENT

Treatment will depend on the cause of your symptom. Be sure to tell your doctor if you are taking any medications (including birth control pills), if you have any kidney disease in your family, and whether or not you have been exercising strenuously. Also, if your job is industrial, it will be important to know whether you have been exposed to gold, mercury, or hydrocarbons since these substances can damage your kidneys. After his examination, your doctor will need to do a urinalysis to determine if blood is present. If he suspects an infection, he'll order a culture and begin antibiotic therapy. If he suspects that you are passing a kidney stone, he may request special studies, including X-rays of your kidneys.

CALL YOUR DOCTOR WHEN:

• you think you have blood in your urine.

LOSS OF BLADDER CONTROL (INCONTINENCE)

DESCRIPTION

Loss of bladder control (incontinence) may stem from any of several causes. A bladder infection may make you feel you have to get to the bathroom quickly to avoid losing urine on the way (urge incontinence). A defect or weakness in the muscles controlling your bladder function can also cause incontinence, in which case even mild physical stress such as coughing, laughing, running, or lifting may cause urine to leak (stress incontinence). This is most common in women whose pelvic muscles have become weakened after childbirth. An enlarged prostate gland in an older man may block the flow of urine from the bladder. When the bladder is full, it may leak (overflow incontinence).

WHEN TO BE CONCERNED

An occasional involuntary loss of urine is generally not serious. It can happen to anyone who has put off that visit to the rest room for too long. But, if this symptom persists, call your doctor. Other symptoms such as burning, frequent urination, or blood in the urine indicate a need for medical evaluation.

TREATMENT

Whenever you experience incontinence, your doctor will want to determine the cause. Infections are usually treated with antibiotics (see Frequent Urination). Women with weakness in the muscles controlling the bladder may benefit from special exercises (Kegel exercises) to strengthen these muscles. Follow your doctor's instructions. If the exercises are not successful, surgical correction may be necessary. Men with enlarged prostate glands may also require surgery.

CALL YOUR DOCTOR WHEN:

• you experience incontinence that persists.

BED-WETTING

DESCRIPTION

Involuntary, persistent bed-wetting during sleep is abnormal beyond age five or six. For some reasons, this symptom is more common in boys than in girls and often runs in families. The cause may be emotional, especially if you've been too insistent on toilet training before your child was ready. If your child sleeps especially soundly, he may not wake up when his bladder is full. Abnormalities of the urinary tract, infections, epilepsy, and diabetes also may cause bed-wetting.

WHEN TO BE CONCERNED

Every child will develop at a different speed. Don't be alarmed if your child takes slightly longer than another child to become toilet-trained. However, if the child is over five or six or has been toilet-trained and suddenly starts bed-wetting, consult your physician.

TREATMENT

One way to prevent the emotional problems that may cause bed-wetting is to recognize when your child is ready for toilet training. He must be able to carry out simple verbal commands. Signs of readiness include dry periods that last several hours as well as interest in sitting on the toilet or getting changed when wet.

Never force your child. If he continues to resist, postpone training for a few weeks. When you start again, try behavior modification techniques. Reinforce use of the toilet by giving rewards. Once a pattern is established, gradually withdraw these rewards. If this is unsuccessful, consult your physician.

If your child has been toilet-trained and suddenly starts bed-wetting, your doctor will want to evaluate his urinary system, particularly when there are no apparent emotional problems. Besides a complete physical examination and urinalysis, he may order special X-rays.

Infections are treated with antibiotics. Occasionally, certain abnormalities of the urinary tract will require surgery. If your child is a deep sleeper, your doctor may recommend medication and/or a conditioning device in which a small amount of urine sets off an alarm.

CALL YOUR DOCTOR WHEN:

• your child begins bed-wetting after successful toilet training.

Chapter 13

Symptoms and Diseases of the Female Organs

MENSTRUAL IRREGULARITY

DESCRIPTION

You probably think of menstruation as just your monthly flow. But the fact is, bleeding is actually the end of a cycle that lasts an average of 28 days (*see* Facts about Menstruation).

Menstruation varies from woman to woman. While the average length of the menstrual cycle is 28 days, some women menstruate every 21 days, others every 36 days. And it is not necessarily abnormal for you to skip a period once in a while. Travel, emotional upset, or illness can temporarily interrupt your cycle. Typically, women taking birth control pills miss occasional periods.

A missed period is also one of the first signs of pregnancy (*see* Signs of Pregnancy), but not always. Some women have "false" periods and bleed even though they are pregnant. In fact, two or three periods in early pregnancy is not unheard of. Unpredictable periods are very common among teenagers whose periods have just begun. If you are over 45, skipped periods may be the first signal of the coming change of life (*see* Changes with Menopause).

What about bleeding between periods? About 10 percent of women have "spotting" or light bleeding for a day or two around the time when an egg is released from the ovary (ovulation). Mid-cycle bleeding is harmless. If this is the cause of your bleeding, your next period should begin exactly 14 days later.

Just as the regularity of cycles may vary among women, so does the amount of bleeding with each period. If you are average, you bleed for three to seven days and lose about 8–10 tablespoons of blood and tissue. Some women have a heavy flow of blood, while some have a very light flow. Sometimes the blood is bright red; sometimes it is dark brown. Some women start with a heavy flow, and then the bleeding slows down. Others start off with spotting and then develop heavier bleeding. All of this is normal.

WHEN TO BE CONCERNED

Anytime the pattern of your bleeding changes, consult your physician. Irregular, unpredictable bleeding has many causes, including uterine infection, fibroid tumors (*see* Menstrual Cramps), thyroid disease, an IUD, birth control pills, and tubal pregnancy. If you are over 30, your doctor will need to check you for uterine or cervical cancer. If you have gone through menopause (no periods for at least six months), report even the tiniest trace of bleeding.

Unusually heavy bleeding accounts for at least half of all irregular bleeding problems. Generally, it is not serious unless you lose so much blood that you become anemic. Your doctor should make that determination with blood tests. Symptoms may vary from none to severe shortness of breath. Call your doctor if your periods are unusually heavy.

If you have missed a period, the rule to remember is that pregnant women don't always miss periods and missed periods don't always signal pregnancy. See your doctor.

TREATMENT

In order to determine the cause of your irregular periods, your doctor will need to do a complete examination, including a pelvic exam. If the cause of your abnormal periods is a temporary hormone imbalance, your problem is likely to resolve itself without treatment.

However, if you have a specific problem such as an infection, a fibroid tumor, or a more serious hormone imbalance, your doctor will advise appropriate therapy. If you are over 30 or there is any question about the cause of your bleeding, he may suggest a surgical procedure known as a D & C to be sure you don't have uterine cancer.

If you are of childbearing age and have missed a period, a pregnancy test will be the first step in your evaluation. If you're taking birth control pills and haven't forgotten any, your doctor may advise you to continue your regular pill schedule for the next cycle. If you have missed a pill or two or have any signs of pregnancy in addition to your missed period, stop your pills, use another method of birth control, and have a pregnancy test and exam promptly.

CALL YOUR DOCTOR WHEN:

- the pattern of your bleeding changes.
- you miss a period and think you may be pregnant.
- you have gone through menopause and begin bleeding again.
- your periods are unusually heavy.

FACTS ABOUT MENSTRUATION

- Menstruation usually starts about 2½ years after breast tissue begins to develop.
- In the United States, menstruation begins at an average age of 12.6 years.
- For the first 12–18 months, menstrual cycles usually occur without ovulation (anovulatory).
- A normal menstrual cycle may be between 21 and 36 days.
- The average menstrual period lasts between 3 and 7 days.
- During an average period, blood loss is between 8 and 10 tablespoons.
- A pad or tampon absorbs between 1 and 2 tablespoons.
- Menstrual blood does not normally clot.

SIGNS OF PREGNANCY
(FIRST 6–12 WEEKS)

- missed period
- frequent urination (waking up at night to urinate)
- breast tenderness and swelling
- queasiness or nausea (especially sensitivity to smells)
- gagging and/or vomiting
- unusual food cravings (especially ice, clay, or cornstarch—may indicate iron deficiency)
- fatigue
- faintness
- weight gain
- fullness in the lower abdomen
- increased vaginal discharge
- mood swings (possibly increased interest in sex)
- improved or worsened complexion

POSSIBLE CHANGES WITH MENOPAUSE

Premenopause
(Usually Six Months to Two Years)

- skipped periods
- decreased menstrual bleeding
- heavier than normal menstrual bleeding
- sleep disruption and night sweats
- hot flashes

Postmenopause

- no periods for at least six consecutive months
- vaginal dryness and itching (may cause painful intercourse)
- thinning of bones (osteoporosis)
- gain in weight
- possible increase in body and facial hair

MENSTRUAL CRAMPS

DESCRIPTION

Cramping just before or during their menstrual periods (dysmenor-rhea) is a common and unpleasant symptom for many women. For some, this is so severe that once a month they may have to take time off from work or school. Occasionally, there is associated passage of large clots.

When this pattern occurs within a year after you have your first period, it is called primary dysmenorrhea. Some experts think this pain is due to contractions of the uterus, probably caused by a substance it produces called prostaglandin. This is the most common type of menstrual cramping and, while painful, is generally not associated with any abnormalities in the female reproductive system.

On the other hand, women who develop severe cramping after years of relatively comfortable periods may have secondary dysmenor-rhea. In these cases, there is generally an underlying problem such as chronic pelvic infections (*see* Cervical Pain), endometriosis, or fibroid tumors that require specific treatment.

Endometriosis is a condition in which tissue that normally lines the uterus is found in other parts of your body, including your ovaries. No one knows the cause, but it seems to occur in women in their 30s and 40s who have delayed having children.

Fibroid tumors are benign (not cancerous) growths of fibrous and muscle tissue that develop in the wall of the uterus, usually in women over 30.

WHEN TO BE CONCERNED

With new drugs available, the cramping with primary dysmenor-rhea can generally be controlled. However, if you are so disabled by the pain that you can't function normally, or if you have secondary dysmenorrhea (pain-free periods for years and then severe cramps), consult your physician.

TREATMENT

Because the cramping in primary dysmenorrhea may be related to prostaglandin effects on the uterus, it is now felt that certain drugs that have antiprostaglandin properties may work to relieve your cramping. Aspirin is one of these drugs. Another is a new drug called ibuprofen (Advil, Nuprin), which you can also buy in any pharmacy. If you are not allergic to aspirin and have no ulcer disease, try this before consulting your physician. Read the label and take only as directed.

If your cramping becomes so severe that home treatment is not effective, a complete examination by your physician is indicated. If you have an infection, he will prescribe appropriate therapy. If you have endometriosis, treatment will depend on many factors, including your age, the severity of your symptoms, and your desire to have children. That's because pregnancy as well as menopause seems to improve the course of this disorder. Sometimes hormone treatments or surgery may relieve your symptoms. Only in very severe cases should a hysterectomy be necessary.

There is no medication for fibroid tumors. If they are small, your doctor will simply check you regularly. If they become very large or if your bleeding is so heavy that you become anemic, he may suggest surgery.

CALL YOUR DOCTOR WHEN:

- you have such severe menstrual cramps that you are unable to function normally and home therapy is not effective.

PREMENSTRUAL SYNDROME

DESCRIPTION

It has been estimated that between 40 and 90 percent of all women suffer from symptoms of premenstrual syndrome (PMS). Yet, until only recently, it was not recognized as a genuine physical problem. Today, while the cause is still uncertain, many theories are being studied. Some scientists feel there may be a malfunction in the production of hormones during the menstrual cycle, especially a hormone called progesterone. Others are looking into a link between the unpleasant symptoms of PMS and nutritional and/or chemical deficiencies such as hypoglycemia and a lack of vitamin B_6. Because of the fact that there are so many symptoms associated with PMS, it is even possible that there is more than one cause.

Women who have this condition complain of feeling irritable, nervous, and/or depressed. They may also develop food cravings (especially for sweets), fatigue, general aches and pains, headaches, abdominal bloating, breast tenderness, and water retention. For some, the symptoms are only a slight inconvenience, causing two or three days of mild discomfort. But for more than a third, the symptoms are more severe and may last a few days to two weeks before every period.

If you suffer from PMS, your symptoms may not be exactly the same as those of another woman who has it. That's because *how* PMS affects you seems to depend on your particular physical makeup, personality, and circumstances. What does seem to be true for all women is that their symptoms follow a more or less regular pattern, occurring at the same time each month. Typically all these symptoms disappear shortly after menstruation begins.

WHEN TO BE CONCERNED

Most women can cope with the milder symptoms of PMS, but for others the physical and behavioral symptoms are intolerable. If your symptoms are disrupting your life, consult your doctor.

TREATMENT

First, you need to determine if you actually have premenstrual syndrome. One of the easiest ways to do so is to chart when your symptoms occur to see if there is a regular pattern each month—symptoms during the week or 10 days before your period and no symptoms the rest of the time.

Once you have determined that you definitely suffer from PMS, there are some things you can do for yourself before seeking medical attention. Try to reduce any expected stress when PMS is due (*see* Positive Health Care, Part I). In general, avoid situations that will tax you.

If you have aches and pains, a hot water bottle applied to the affected area can be soothing. Massaging aching muscles may also help. Some women find relief in taking a hot bath and then lying down for a while. Hot drinks such as herb tea and soup will warm and comfort you. Herb tea has the added advantage of being a natural diuretic if you suffer from water retention.

If you feel you need medication for your menstrual cramps, try either aspirin or ibuprofen (Advil, Nuprin), sold at any pharmacy. Follow the directions on the bottle.

Some women report that changing dietary habits relieves their PMS symptoms. Limit consumption of refined sugar, salt, caffeine, red meat, and alcohol. Increase your intake of complex carbohydrates (whole grains, potatoes, pasta, for example). It can take three to six months to achieve maximum results with this approach, so be patient.

Once you've tried home remedies without success, it's time to consult your doctor. A thorough physical examination, including a pelvic exam, is an important first step in order to be sure you don't have any other medical or psychological problem. Don't forget to bring your symptom chart with you. This record will be extremely helpful to your gynecologist in making the diagnosis.

Because research on PMS is quite new, treatment is still not uniform. Your doctor will try to tailor your treatment to your individual symptoms, probably recommending special diets and/or medication. If you have problems with fluid retention, he may prescribe fluid pills (diuretics). Some physicians believe pyridoxine (vitamin B_6) is useful. Others prefer progesterone therapy.

Finally, remember that PMS is not "all in your mind." For many women, just knowing that this is a temporary physical condition is reassuring.

CALL YOUR DOCTOR WHEN:

- you believe you are suffering from PMS and have tried home remedies without success.

VAGINAL DISCHARGE AND ITCHING

DESCRIPTION

Vaginal discharge is probably one of the most common complaints among women. Between TV and popular magazines, women have been convinced that any discharge is abnormal and requires, at the very least, self-treatment with a scented douche or feminine hygiene spray. Frequently, the fear is that this represents a venereal disease or even cancer.

The fact is, a certain amount of discharge from the vagina is normal during the reproductive years. Outer cells from the cervix and vagina are constantly being shed in the form of a small amount of white or grayish-white material. Birth control pills and pregnancy may increase the discharge. Likewise, with sexual stimulation, the cervix and a pair of glands located at the junction of the vagina and vulva (Bartholin's glands) secrete a watery or mucuslike substance. Blood-tinged discharge may appear just around the time of ovulation.

To summarize: normal vaginal discharges are generally small in amount, white or clear, and nonbloody (except around ovulation). There is no particular odor and no itching or irritation. So when is a discharge abnormal? When you notice a thick white or yellow discharge that produces itching, pain, irritation, and/or an unpleasant odor, you may have an infection, usually of the vagina and/or cervix (*see* Cervical Pain).

Candida albicans (Monilia), or yeast, is the most common cause of vaginal infections. Although yeast is normally present in the vagina, changes in vaginal chemistry may allow these organisms to multiply.

If you are taking certain antibiotics or birth control pills, or if you are pregnant or have diabetes, you may have an increased risk of developing a yeast infection. Typically, the discharge will be thick and white, almost like cottage cheese. You may experience intense itching at the vaginal opening as well as burning during urination and/or intercourse.

Trichomonas is a type of parasitic organism that produces a greenish-yellow, foamy vaginal discharge, often associated with an unpleasant odor. Itching and inflammation are also common. Trichomonas can be transmitted through sexual contact.

A third common vaginal infection that produces discharge and itching is caused by bacteria (non-specific vaginitis). Like Trichomonas, it can be transmitted through intercourse.

WHEN TO BE CONCERNED

Vaginal discharge does not necessarily indicate infection or any other serious problem requiring treatment. If your only symptom is the discharge, unless you are very uncomfortable, there is probably no cause for concern. It is only when the discharge is irritating and associated with itching and/or unpleasant odor that you need to consult your physician.

TREATMENT

You may have heard that douching either prevents infection or should be used to treat any discharge. Actually, douching is not necessary for routine or normal feminine hygiene. It's possible to live your whole life in good health without douching. A certain amount of yeast and bacteria are normally present in the vagina, and douching too frequently may actually disturb that balance. If you feel cleaner douching, do so no more than two to four times per month. A simple mixture of one ounce of white vinegar to one quart of water is adequate. Perfumed douches or deodorant hygiene sprays may actually produce local irritation.

If your discharge is irritating and/or associated with itching, make an appointment with your doctor. Be sure to tell him if you are taking any antibiotics or birth control pills, if you are diabetic, or if you think you may be pregnant. He can confirm the diagnosis of infection by looking at the discharge under a microscope.

Vaginal medications are usually prescribed for yeast infections, oral medications for Trichomonas and bacterial vaginitis. Your doctor may suggest treating your sexual partner if you have a Trichomonas or bacterial infection. Complete all medication prescribed in order to ensure a complete cure. If vaginal medication is prescribed, tampons should probably not be used during treatment, since they will absorb the medication, reducing its effectiveness.

CALL YOUR DOCTOR WHEN:

- you have a thick white or yellow vaginal discharge associated with itching, burning, pain, and/or unpleasant odor.

VAGINAL PAIN

DESCRIPTION

Pain around the opening of the vagina can be caused by many different problems. If you have a vaginal infection, you may experience burning, itching, and discharge as well as pain (*see* Vaginal Discharge and Itching). Because inflamed tissue is sensitive to any kind of friction or pressure, you are likely to notice pain soon after intercourse (*see* Painful Intercourse).

Today the herpes virus has become a common source of genital infection. It is transmitted from person to person through genital-genital or oral-genital contact. Symptoms are noticeable two to seven days after you are exposed. Typically, with first infections in women (primary infections), small fluid-filled blisters (vesicles) appear on the vulva and/or cervix (*see* Cervical Pain). These blisters rupture, leaving shallow, painful sores that gradually form a scab over a two- or three-week period. You may experience associated symptoms such as fever, generalized aches and pains, swollen glands, neuralgia (burning or stabbing pain), and headaches.

After this first attack, the virus retreats to nerve clusters alongside the spinal column, where it is beyond the reach of the body's defense system. This stage (latency) can last forever or be broken when the virus is reactivated, reinfecting the original site. Such recurrences may take place as often as twice a month or as rarely as once a decade.

If you do become infected with herpes, you have a one in three chance of experiencing recurrent episodes. Generally, recurrent infections are milder. Just before the sores appear, you may notice a tingling or burning sensation near the site. The sores themselves may burn, itch, or be quite painful. In addition, you may notice burning on urination and/or a vaginal discharge.

Some women experience vaginal pain because they have a sensitivity or allergy to perfumed douches, deodorant feminine hygiene sprays, birth control foam, and/or contraceptive jelly or cream.

Pain deep in the vagina can arise from the cervix, uterus, fallopian tubes, or ovaries or from nearby intestines or bladder. Usually, this kind of pain is associated with painful intercourse.

WHEN TO BE CONCERNED

Any vaginal pain is abnormal, although the cause may be something as simple as a tiny scratch produced by your own fingernail. It can be a devastating problem that interferes with your normal routine, including sexual functioning. If this symptom doesn't go away within a short time or is associated with other symptoms such as painful intercourse, vaginal discharge, sores, burning, and/or itching, see your doctor. Severe abdominal pain with or without fever suggests a serious problem requiring *immediate* attention.

TREATMENT

If you are using a particular vaginal product that you think is causing your symptoms, avoid it for a few days to see if your symptoms go away. If you have scratched yourself, and there is no evidence of infection (pus or discharge), a warm bath may give you relief. Otherwise, see your doctor so that he can identify the cause of your vaginal pain and prescribe appropriate treatment.

In addition to medication available for bacterial, yeast, and Trichomonas infections, today there is an approved drug for the herpes virus. It is called Acyclovir or Zovirax and can be used for both primary and recurrent infections.

While you are being treated, avoid intercourse. Keep the herpes sores clean and dry. Remember, ointments and creams (except those prescribed to treat secondary infections) tend to prolong healing. Avoid scratching, picking, or touching the sores since this transfers the virus to other parts of your body. The only way at present to prevent herpes is to avoid exposure, so don't be afraid to ask a new sexual partner if he or she has genital herpes.

CALL YOUR DOCTOR WHEN:

- you have pain around the opening of the vagina associated with painful intercourse, discharge, sores, itching, and/or burning.
- you have pain deeper in the vagina, especially if there is associated abdominal pain.

CERVICAL PAIN

DESCRIPTION

You can't see your cervix because it is the narrow passage at the lower end of your uterus that connects with your vagina. However, if you were to put your finger inside the vagina, your cervix would feel like the tip of your nose. If you notice pain during intercourse or when you touch your cervix, it is possible you have an inflammation of the cervix (cervicitis).

Inflammation may occur when cervical tissue is invaded by bacteria or other organisms (infection) or by chemicals in vaginal hygiene products. Besides cervical pain, you may experience a large amount of yellow or grayish-white vaginal discharge with a foul odor (*see* Vaginal Discharge and Itching), spotting or bleeding after intercourse, fever, or abdominal and/or back pain.

Bacteria normally found in the vagina can cause cervicitis if they invade the mucous glands in the cervical canal and begin to multiply. However, other bacteria such as gonorrhea and chlamydia are transmitted from one sexual partner to another. In addition to bacteria, yeast, Trichomonas, and herpes (*see* Vaginal Pain) can cause infections of the cervix.

WHEN TO BE CONCERNED

Anytime you experience cervical pain, bleeding with intercourse, or foul vaginal discharge, check with your physician. Untreated cervical infections can spread to other pelvic organs such as your fallopian tubes and ovaries, causing serious complications, including infertility (*see* Infertility).

If you happen to have an infection of the cervix at the time your doctor does a Pap smear, it is possible the test will be reported as abnormal. That's because the inflammation causes abnormal but noncancerous cell changes. Therefore, it is important to have your Pap test repeated when your infection clears up.

TREATMENT

Your physician may suspect cervicitis on the basis of your symptoms, the appearance of your cervix during your pelvic exam (raw, eroded areas), or an abnormal Pap smear. If the diagnosis is an infection, he will prescribe appropriate medication. Those infections like gonorrhea, chlamydia, and Trichomonas require treating your sexual partner as well. Avoid intercourse until treatment is completed. If you have an IUD, your doctor may suggest removing it since the string could be a source of infection.

If a chemical irritant such as a perfumed douche or deodorant feminine hygiene spray is suspected, your doctor will advise you to avoid it. Prolonged or repeated cervicitis may require minor surgery.

CALL YOUR DOCTOR WHEN:

- you experience painful intercourse or pain when you touch your cervix (with or without other symptoms).
- you notice spotting or bleeding after intercourse.
- you have a vaginal discharge associated with a foul odor.

BREAST LUMPS

DESCRIPTION

Many women live in fear of breast cancer. In some ways, there is reason for concern: breast cancer is a leading cause of death among women. However, a lump in your breast doesn't necessarily mean you have cancer. Most lumps are benign (noncancerous).

Experts estimate that over half of all women normally have some lumpiness in their breasts. This is especially true just before menstruation, when hormone changes affect the milk-producing glands of your breasts. Often these lumps are painful and disappear immediately after your period.

If you notice a movable, solid, firm, rubbery, painless lump in your breast, this may also be a benign mass called a fibroadenoma. It is made up of gland cells and fibrous tissue.

Lumps that don't feel solid may have fluid inside (cysts). These are also benign. There is no good evidence to show that women who develop cysts are more likely to develop cancer. Often cysts are found in both breasts and tend to be painful.

WHEN TO BE CONCERNED

If you notice a lump in your breast, the first thing to do is relax. Most breast lumps are not cancer. However, it is important to see your doctor as soon as possible for proper evaluation. Remember, there is absolutely nothing to be gained by waiting.

Don't avoid seeking medical attention just because your lump is painless. Local pain and/or tenderness only rarely accompany malignant breast diseases. If your mother or sister had breast cancer, or if you have put off having children past age 35, your risk of developing breast cancer is greater than that of other women.

TREATMENT

Most breast cancers are first discovered by women themselves. Since breast cancers found early and treated promptly have the best chance for cure, learning how to examine your breasts properly can help save your life (*see* Breast Self-Exam).

The best time to check yourself is once a month, just after your period, when your breasts are less likely to be tender and swollen. If you have gone through menopause, do breast self-examinations on the first day of every month. Your doctor should do a breast exam each time you have a Pap smear (at least every three years from age 20–40 and yearly after age 40).

A mammogram is a low-dose X-ray of the breasts that can help detect cancers too small for you to feel. You should have one between the ages of 35 and 40 as a base line. From 40 to 49, the American Cancer Society recommends one every one to two years, depending on the findings, your family history, and your doctor's advice. After age 50, you should have one yearly.

If you and/or your doctor discovers a lump and it's right *before* your period, he may suggest that you return for a reexamination in two weeks following the end of that period. This is because the lump may simply be related to monthly hormone changes and will disappear by the next visit.

If you have a single lump that your doctor feels is almost certainly a benign fluid-filled cyst, he may suggest aspiration. This is a simple office procedure. After numbing the skin with local anesthesia, he'll use a small needle to remove the fluid. The lump should completely disappear. In some cases, your doctor will first order a test called an ultrasound. This is a painless sound wave examination of the breast that helps to distinguish solid masses from cysts.

If there is any question at all about your lump, especially if you are over 30, your doctor will probably first order a mammogram and then recommend a biopsy. This can be done on an outpatient basis.

If the result is positive for cancer, treatment will depend on the extent of the disease and your age. Today not every woman with breast cancer needs to have the breast removed (mastectomy). In some cases, just removing the lump (lumpectomy) with or without additional drug or radiation therapy may be sufficient. However, your doctor should discuss all the treatment options with you. Listen carefully and ask questions.

CALL YOUR DOCTOR WHEN:

• you feel a breast lump (even if there's no pain).

BREAST SELF-EXAM

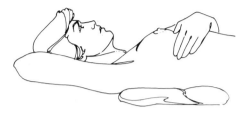 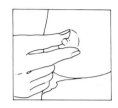

Lying Down

Lie down flat on your back with a pillow under your right shoulder and your right hand behind your head. With the fingertips of your left hand flat, gently press against your right breast, using a circular motion. Begin at the outermost part of your breast (near your armpit). Check for lumps, hard knots, or thickenings. When the first circle is completed, start again about one inch inward. Repeat the circles, moving in toward the nipple until your entire breast has been covered. Then do the same examination of your left breast. Finally, squeeze each nipple gently between thumb and index finger and look for any discharge.

Sitting or Standing

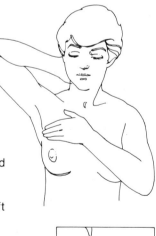

Inspect your breasts while sitting or standing in front of a mirror. First check with your hands on your hips and muscles tensed. Remember, most women have one breast larger than the other and even higher than the other. Look for any changes, including swelling, indentation or dimpling of the skin, or retraction of the nipples. Do the same examination with your arms raised above your head. Next, with your right arm behind your head, take your left hand and examine your right breast using the same technique you used lying down. When you are done, examine your left breast using your right hand with your left arm behind your head. This examination can be done in the shower or bath.

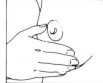

NIPPLE DISCHARGE

DESCRIPTION

If you notice a discharge from your nipples, don't panic. Some women have a clear or milky nipple secretion during pregnancy or after a delivery (especially when nursing), a miscarriage, or an abortion. Also, certain drugs, including marijuana, birth control pills, and estrogen (for menopausal symptoms) may sometimes cause a slight nipple discharge. Women whose sexual patterns include a great deal of breast stimulation may also develop a nipple discharge.

WHEN TO BE CONCERNED

Although a nipple discharge may be normal, you should always consult your physician if you experience this symptom (whether the discharge is clear, pus-filled, or bloody). Besides cancer, a discharge may be caused by infection in your breast or certain diseases that affect hormone levels in your body.

TREATMENT

Your doctor will do a careful breast examination to check for any lumps that may be present in addition to the nipple discharge. Remember to tell him if you are taking any drugs since they could be causing your discharge. Depending on his findings, he may suggest a mammogram and possibly a biopsy. He may collect samples of the discharge to be tested for cancer cells. If he suspects a disease affecting your hormone levels, he will probably order special blood and urine tests. If your problem is an infection, he'll prescribe appropriate antibiotics, with or without minor surgery.

CALL YOUR DOCTOR WHEN:

• you notice any discharge from one or both nipples.

PAINFUL INTERCOURSE

DESCRIPTION

Painful intercourse is a symptom with both physical and psychological causes. Two of the most common physical causes are friction against vaginal tissue inflamed from infection or irritation (*see* Vaginal Pain) and friction against dry, poorly lubricated vaginal tissue.

If you and your partner engage in intercourse before you are fully aroused, your vagina may not be moistened completely. Normally, vaginal lubrication is one response to sexual arousal. This response may be decreased by certain medications such as antihistamines or by low estrogen levels following pregnancy (especially if you are nursing) and after menopause (*see* Changes with Menopause).

Pain deep in the vagina during intercourse may be the first sign of a cervical infection (*see* Cervical Pain), although the symptom may arise from the uterus, tubes, or ovaries or from nearby intestines or bladder.

Some women who experience painful intercourse have spasms of the vaginal muscles. They may have the same symptom during a pelvic examination. The cause is generally psychological, often the result of a past unpleasant sexual experience.

WHEN TO BE CONCERNED

Because painful intercourse is often the first sign of infection or other physical problem, consult your doctor. If you have associated severe abdominal pain, with or without fever, seek *immediate* attention.

TREATMENT

If you know your problem is insufficient arousal during intercourse, allowing time for the normal lubrication response may be all you need to do. If you have vaginal dryness, and you've been through menopause, you may want to try extra lubrication during intercourse such as a nonprescription water-soluble lubricant like K-Y jelly.

Estrogen, as either oral pills or vaginal cream, may be helpful, but discuss this with your doctor since estrogen use is still controversial.

If you don't know the cause, see your doctor. Remember to bring any medications you are taking, since they could be the problem. If you have an infection, the proper medication will relieve your symptoms.

If you have painful spasm of your vaginal muscles, your doctor may recommend counseling and conditioning exercises that you can do at home. Pain or muscle tightness severe enough to make intercourse impossible is unusual, but even this generally resolves with treatment. If your doctor determines that the problem is a small opening in the membrane (hymen) covering the vagina, he may recommend exercises that you can do at home and, in extreme cases, minor surgery.

CALL YOUR DOCTOR WHEN:

• you experience repeated painful intercourse, with or without other symptoms.

INFERTILITY

DESCRIPTION

About 10-15 percent of all couples have trouble conceiving, and the problem is just as likely to be the male partner's as the female's. Male infertility is commonly caused by problems with sperm (low count, abnormal shape or motion) although abnormalities of the urethra, testicle (see Scrotal Masses), and/or penis may also be responsible. Female infertility may stem from nutritional deficiencies, hormone imbalance, infections (see Cervical Pain), tumors, or other abnormalities in the reproductive organs. Often a couple's infertility is the result of a combination of these factors.

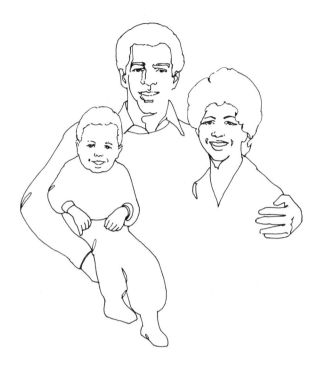

WHEN TO BE CONCERNED

Generally, you shouldn't even concern yourself with infertility until you've tried to conceive for at least a year. However, women who've had several miscarriages or menstruate irregularly may have difficulty getting pregnant without treatment. Likewise, see your physician early if the male partner had mumps after childhood that affected his testicles.

TREATMENT

If you want to become pregnant for the first time and you've been trying for less than a year, relax. Stress itself can contribute to fertility problems. Keep a careful record of your menstrual cycles, including taking your temperature each morning as soon as you wake up (basal body temperature). There will be a slight drop and then rise (less than one degree) when you ovulate (day 14 if you have a 28-day cycle).

Your fertile period is about two days before and two days after ovulation. Have intercourse three or four times during this time. Avoid douching and don't use lubricants on or before your fertile days since this may kill sperm. If you were taking birth control pills and stopped, it may take up to six months before you become pregnant, so don't panic.

Once you decide to consult your physician, it will take about three months for both partners to be thoroughly evaluated and the cause of infertility determined. Be prepared to answer many detailed and personal questions such as frequency and position of intercourse, sexual techniques, history of venereal disease, and/or abortions. Don't be embarrassed. It's important to be honest with your doctor.

After a complete physical examination, your physician will probably order certain blood and urine tests. Special tests for the female partner may be necessary, including checking to be sure there is no blockage of the tubes. Semen analysis is also a routine part of every fertility evaluation.

Once your doctor determines the cause of your infertility, he will recommend specific therapy. Today, there are many new approaches to treatment, so be hopeful. There is an excellent chance that you will be able to have that baby you want.

CALL YOUR DOCTOR WHEN:

* you have tried to become pregnant for one year without success unless the male partner had mumps involving the testicles or the female has already had several miscarriages. With these situations, you need not wait one year before seeing your doctor.

Chapter 14

Symptoms and Diseases of the Male Organs

PENILE DISCHARGE

DESCRIPTION

The penis serves a vital function for two entirely separate organ systems. The urethra, the tube from the bladder that runs through the penis, is vital to both your urinary and reproductive systems. A discharge from your urethra is a common symptom often caused by inflammation of this tube itself or by an infection in your prostate.

An inflammation of the tube itself, called urethritis, most commonly causes a penile discharge. This inflammation is usually caused by a sexually transmitted infection but may rarely occur from trauma as well as certain foods or medications. In the past, most sexually transmitted infections were due to gonorrhea, but now an organism called chlamydia is even more common.

If you have gonorrhea, your discharge will be a thick greenish-yellow. If your discharge is watery-white, it is most likely due to chlamydia. A third organism, also transmitted sexually, that often causes a penile discharge with itching is called Trichomonas. Other symptoms, besides a discharge, caused by these infections may include itching, pain in the head (glans) of the penis, pain in the testicles, and painful urination (*see* Burning on Urination).

The prostate gland lies below the bladder, surrounding the urethra. Infections of the prostate can also lead to urethritis and penile discharge. Acute prostatitis is usually seen in younger men and is often caused by sexually transmitted infections. Other symptoms of acute prostatitis besides urethral discharge are pain radiating to the testicles; fever; and difficult, frequent, burning urination. Chronic prostatitis is more common in older men than in younger men and rarely results from an infection. Symptoms of back pain and urinary obstruction, rather than penile discharge, are usually present.

WHEN TO BE CONCERNED

Any discharge from your penis is abnormal and should be checked by your doctor. If you are very active sexually, a sexually transmitted infection is most likely. If you've been drinking heavily or are taking any new medications or vitamins, these may rarely cause a slight irritation and a scanty discharge. Some experts even believe that these symptoms can have a psychosomatic cause based on guilt feelings following sexual intercourse.

Prostatitis results from a urethral infection or from an infection carried through the bloodstream. If you have a fever, urinary symptoms, or pain in your testicles or low back, with or without a penile discharge, suspect prostatitis.

TREATMENT

Any penile discharge that lasts more than a day or two, even without other symptoms, requires a medical evaluation. Your doctor will take a careful history and probably look at your discharge under a microscope. He may also request a culture to confirm his diagnosis. If you have an infection, he'll prescribe antibiotics. Your sexual partner should be checked and treated at the same time. If your penile discharge stems from acute prostatitis, it will also need to be cultured to determine the cause of infection. Again, your sexual partner should be examined and treated. Drink lots of fluids, but avoid alcohol and sexual intercourse until your condition has cleared up.

Chronic prostatitis and an enlarged prostate causing urinary obstruction may require surgical treatment. Older men should have annual rectal and prostate examinations, even in the absence of symptoms, as part of a regular program of cancer screening.

CALL YOUR DOCTOR WHEN:

- you have any penile discharge, with or without other symptoms.
- you have any symptoms of testicular or low back pain with difficulty urinating.

PENILE PAIN

DESCRIPTION

Penile pain is most commonly caused by an infection in the tube known as the urethra, which leads from the bladder through the penis. These infections commonly cause pain in the penis and a discharge (*see* Penile Discharge). Two other common causes of penile pain are trauma to the penis, usually from intercourse, and blisters or ulcerations on the head (glans) or shaft of the penis itself.

Any irritation or ulceration of the skin of the penis requires a careful medical evaluation. Genital herpes (type II) is a viral infection spread by sexual contact that has reached almost epidemic proportions. It is easily the most common cause of ulceration of the penis. Seven to 10 days after contact, small blisters (vesicles) usually develop on the glans or shaft of the penis. These blisters usually break open and become small superficial ulcers. The lymph nodes in your groin may become enlarged and tender.

Most people realize that syphilis is a serious disease. The problem is that many fail to recognize it because the ulcer (chancre) that it causes is often painless. The ulcer usually appears within four weeks of infection and heals by itself within another four to eight weeks. The lymph nodes in your groin may become enlarged, but they're usually not tender. Failure to diagnose and treat this infection promptly can result in serious long-term consequences.

WHEN TO BE CONCERNED

Any ulceration on your penis should be a cause for concern, regardless of whether or not it is painful. Both genital herpes and syphilis, as well as other infections, may cause swelling and/or tenderness in your groin. Also, if any open ulcer is not kept scrupulously clean, you may develop a secondary bacterial infection.

TREATMENT

Mild trauma to the penis is usually relieved by brief abstinence from sexual activity. Any penile blisters or ulcerations require prompt diagnosis and treatment. Do not try home remedies or off-the-shelf ointments. If your doctor suspects herpes, he may culture the ulcer to confirm his diagnosis. There is a recently approved topical and oral medication for herpes (Acyclovir or Zovirax) that your doctor may prescribe. Your sexual partner should be advised of your infection and checked carefully. Avoid further sexual contact while you have any signs of the ulceration. Also, it is most important that you avoid touching your eyes after touching your penis. The herpes virus is highly contagious and causes serious eye infections.

If you have a single penile ulcer that is painless, suspect syphilis. This can usually be diagnosed by several different laboratory tests. If you have early or primary syphilis, your doctor will prescribe penicillin or another antibiotic. Your sexual partner should also be notified and checked. Careful medical follow-up care is important to prevent later complications.

CALL YOUR DOCTOR WHEN:

- you have any penile pain.
- you notice any ulceration or blister on your penis, whether or not it is painful.

PAINFUL URINATION

DESCRIPTION

Painful urination in younger men is most commonly caused by urethritis (*see* Penile Discharge) or cystitis (*see* Burning on Urination). In older men, an enlarged prostate with chronic prostatitis may often cause urinary obstruction with cystitis and frequent urination (*see* Frequent Urination). Also, any blisters or ulcerations (*see* Penile Pain) on the head of your penis near the opening of the urethra can cause painful urination. Kidney stones may cause blood in your urine (*see* Blood in the Urine) and painful urination.

WHEN TO BE CONCERNED

Generally, if you are having any pain when you urinate, with or without any of the above symptoms, schedule a prompt medical evaluation. With some conditions, such as kidney stones, your symptoms may come and go. Don't delay medical care because you think things might improve. Many simple problems can lead to complications if they are not treated promptly.

TREATMENT

Generally, the treatment of pain on urination will depend on your doctor's determination of the underlying cause of your symptoms.

CALL YOUR DOCTOR WHEN:

• you experience any painful urination.

PAIN IN THE TESTICLES

DESCRIPTION

The testicles produce not only sperm, they also produce male hormones. Once sperm are produced, they move into each epididymis (ductlike structures on the top and sides of each testicle). From here, sperm are directed through the spermatic duct (vas deferens) to the penis.

Testicular pain usually commands your attention because of its severity and can result from several conditions. Direct trauma causes severe pain and sometimes a twisting (torsion) of the testicle, cutting off its blood supply. An inguinal hernia, or one related to the groin, also causes pain and swelling on one or both sides of the scrotum and may mimic actual testicular pain. Testicular tumors may also cause pain (*see* Scrotal Masses).

Also, each testicle and epididymis can become infected. Inflammation of the testicles (orchitis) is usually due to infection (often from mumps in men beyond puberty) or follows direct injury. The epididymis may become infected from a sexually transmitted disease or from an infected prostate. Both the testicle and epididymis may become infected together.

Both infections cause symptoms of pain, swelling, fever, and vomiting.

WHEN TO BE CONCERNED

Any testicular trauma that causes pain or swelling should be checked promptly. Any infection of the testicles or epididymis likewise needs prompt treatment. If you feel pain and a mass in your scrotum that gets worse when you cough, suspect an inguinal hernia and seek *immediate* medical evaluation. Any other mass in your scrotum, even if it is painless, requires prompt evaluation.

TREATMENT

If your doctor finds no serious injury, direct trauma to your testicles may be treated with painkillers and cold packs. If you have an inguinal hernia, he'll likely recommend surgery; emergency is called for if it is "strangulated." For infection of the testicles or epididymis, antibiotics, painkillers, cold packs, bed rest, and scrotal support are the mainstays of treatment. Treatment of testicular masses depends on the particular diagnosis.

CALL YOUR DOCTOR WHEN:

- you have any pain in your testicles.

SCROTAL MASSES

DESCRIPTION

Any mass in the scrotum (testicular sac) requires careful medical evaluation. The problem is that most masses, even those that are serious, go undetected because few men examine themselves carefully. This is especially important if you are under age 35, because testicular cancer most commonly occurs between the ages of 15 and 35. While many solid tumors of the testicle itself are often malignant, fortunately, most masses in the scrotum are benign cystic swellings of little significance.

For example, occasionally a collection of fluid (hydrocele) may develop around the testicle, but this usually disappears by itself. Sometimes semen may form a cyst (spermatocele) in the epididymis. A small clump of varicose veins (varicocele) may also feel like a lump in the scrotum, and occasionally these veins may cause infertility.

Solid masses coming from the testicle itself are more likely to be tumors, and these require careful evaluation. In men under 30, testicular tumors are probably the most common solid malignancy.

WHEN TO BE CONCERNED

Generally, any scrotal mass should concern you until it has been checked. Although malignant tumors may cause pain, don't be reassured because a mass is painless or small. Also, don't wait to see if it goes away by itself. Tumors of the testicles themselves are often malignant, and any delay in their diagnosis or treatment may be life-threatening.

TESTICULAR SELF-EXAM

Testicular cancer most commonly occurs in young men 15–35 years of age and early diagnosis and treatment can be lifesaving. If you have had undescended testicles, you are probably at an even greater risk of developing a tumor. Suspicious masses can be detected early if you learn to examine yourself regularly, about once a month.

Your testicles are located behind your penis and within the scrotal sac. They should feel smooth, rubbery, and egg-shaped. Both of your testicles should be of about equal size, with the left sometimes hanging somewhat lower than the right. Your testicles produce both sperm and the male hormone testosterone. The epididymis is a soft collection of tubes behind each testicle that collects the sperm. During ejaculation, the sperm travel through the spermatic duct (vas deferens) to the prostate and out the urethra.

The American Cancer Society recommends the following evaluation:

1. Examine the testicles during or after a hot shower when the heat causes the testicles to drop down and the scrotum to relax.

2. Examine each testicle with a gentle, firm, rolling motion of the testes held between the fingers and thumbs of both hands.

3. Feel for any irregularity on the surface of the testes. Also feel for hardness or swelling or a difference in size between the two.

4. The epididymis can be felt along the top edge of the testes toward the back.

5. Report any unusual lump, firmness, or swelling to your physician right away.

TREATMENT

Early diagnosis as a result of your regular testicular self-exam (*see* Testicular Self-Exam) is most important. Any scrotal mass requires prompt evaluation by your doctor. It is important that he determine whether it originates in the testicle itself or in the surrounding tissues. Most masses that come from the surrounding tissues and are cystic rather than solid can usually be followed medically. Those that originate in the testicle itself and are solid are very likely to be malignant. Various diagnostic procedures are available, and highly suspicious cases may require surgical exploration and biopsy.

CALL YOUR DOCTOR WHEN

• you detect any scrotal mass during your periodic examination.

IMPOTENCE

DESCRIPTION

The problem of impotence is more common than you probably realize, especially in men over 40, and should never be a cause of embarrassment. For years, this inability to achieve and maintain an erection was almost always considered to be due to emotional problems. Often impotence will be temporary, and in many of these cases it may result from stress or another emotional problem. But experts now realize that, in many cases, physical problems also cause impotence.

For example, a decrease in testosterone production may cause this symptom. Since an erection is accomplished when the penis becomes engorged with blood, any condition that narrows or obstructs the arteries to the penis can also cause impotence, including atherosclerosis and pelvic tumors that can obstruct an artery. Similarly, conditions that affect the nerves to the penis may also cause this symptom. Finally, alcohol and many drugs, especially some of those used to treat high blood pressure, have been shown to cause impotence. It is important to remember that this symptom has nothing to do with your interest in sex or your actual fertility.

WHEN TO BE CONCERNED

If you notice that you are suddenly unable to have or sustain an erection, or your impotence has come on gradually, you should seek medical attention as soon as possible. Do not be embarrassed and automatically blame your emotions. Your problem may be a symptom of a serious underlying condition.

TREATMENT

Your treatment will depend on the cause of impotence. After a careful history, your doctor may suggest blood tests to check your testosterone level and other tests to evaluate the circulation to your penis. If he is unable to uncover a physical cause for your symptoms, he may suggest some psychological evaluation and counseling.

CALL YOUR DOCTOR WHEN:

• you are unable to achieve an erection or satisfactorily maintain it to achieve intercourse.

PART IV

SYMPTOMS AND DISEASES OF CHILDREN

Chapter 15

Childhood Concerns

DIARRHEA IN CHILDREN

DESCRIPTION

Ordinarily, you expect your infant or young child to have an occasional loose stool. But since infants and small children can get seriously dehydrated in just a few hours, diarrhea requires prompt evaluation. Complications of diarrhea vary with the degree of dehydration, the child's age and prior health, and other associated symptoms. Besides rapid fluid loss, diarrhea may also quickly lead to a serious salt imbalance.

In an otherwise healthy child, there are many causes of sudden diarrhea. Most common is recent antibiotic treatment for an unrelated problem. Consult your child's doctor about stopping these drugs. Other infections, often in the urinary or respiratory system, also often cause diarrhea in infants and young children. Finally, dietary changes, such as overfeeding a colicky child or introducing new foods, may bring on diarrhea.

WHEN TO BE CONCERNED

Normally, children's bowel habits may vary as much as those of adults. A gradual or sudden change in the consistency or the number of stools or a change in their color to green should concern you. Diarrhea during the first three months of life is especially alarming. Several serious conditions may cause loose stools early on. Likewise, any hint of blood in your child's stool (bright red or tarry black) requires *immediate* care. If the diarrhea is associated with fever, lethargy, or abdominal pain, your child needs *immediate* medical attention.

TREATMENT

Since your young child's diarrhea can rapidly become serious, home treatment for anything but the mildest case is not recommended. Your pediatrician will probably request blood tests to check salt and acid balance and promptly begin to restore fluids, intravenously if necessary. He may have your child fast for a few days until the child's fluid balance improves. After this, he'll begin to search for the underlying cause of the diarrhea. Your child's doctor will likely recommend a diet that is free of protein, milk, and lactose.

CALL YOUR DOCTOR WHEN:

- your infant or young child has more than two loose stools.
- you detect any evidence of bleeding in your child's stools (*call immediately*).
- your child has associated symptoms of fever, lethargy, or abdominal cramps (*call immediately*).

FEVER IN INFANTS AND CHILDREN

DESCRIPTION

As a parent, you should know that fever is one of the most common complaints in any pediatrician's practice. A sudden fever in your infant or young child is most likely caused by an acute infection. Virus infections rarely cause a fever lasting more than 10 days, but untreated or inadequately treated bacterial infections may persist for weeks or months. After two weeks, if no infection or other cause for a fever can be found, other more serious conditions must be considered. This unexplained symptom is called a fever of unknown origin (FUO).

Without other serious symptoms, you can generally assume during the first few days that your child's fever is most likely due to a viral infection. Your doctor can usually diagnose most of these infections by asking some questions, examining your child, and ordering a few laboratory tests. Common childhood viruses include measles, mumps, and chicken pox.

Measles is an acute, highly contagious disease with fever, cough and cold symptoms, mouth lesions, and a generalized rash (*see* Generalized Rashes). Because of recent widespread immunization programs (*see* immunization schedule in Positive Health Care, Part I), outbreaks now usually occur in adolescents, with occasional cases in infants and young children. After one case of measles, your child will have lifelong immunity.

The measles virus usually incubates for one to two weeks before the early symptoms develop. Your child will soon develop characteristic whitish spots (Koplik's spots) on the inside of the cheek within two to four days and a generalized rash a few days later. In severe cases, your child's temperature may reach 104 degrees Fahrenheit and the other symptoms may become severe. There will be characteristic changes in certain routine blood tests.

If your child has a tender swelling under one or both jaws, along with fever and other symptoms of a viral infection, suspect mumps as a likely cause. The mumps virus is usually spread by droplets of infected saliva, but it is generally not as contagious as measles or chicken pox. Most cases usually occur between the ages of 5 and 15, and mumps is extremely rare in children under 2. Beyond puberty, mumps may involve organs other than the salivary glands, particularly the testicles in males (*see* Pain in the Testicles). Recent active immunization programs (*see* immunization schedule in Positive Health Care, Part I) provide immunity to those vaccinated.

After a two- to three-week incubation period, early symptoms of mumps may include headache, tiredness, chills, moderate fever, and finally swollen salivary glands with pain on swallowing. Abdominal pain is a frequent complaint and may indicate inflammation of the pancreas. Mumps usually is self-limited and rarely causes long-term complications.

Chicken pox is primarily a highly contagious disease of childhood. The characteristic symptoms usually occur approximately two weeks after a child has had contact with the disease. Cold symptoms and a mild temperature may begin two or three days before the well-known generalized rash appears. This rash (*see* Generalized Rashes) consists of teardrop-shaped blisters (vesicles) that appear in "crops" and have red borders. As these blisters rupture, crusts form and continue to itch.

Because of the characteristic rash, chicken pox is rarely mistaken for another disease. Complications of chicken pox in children are unusual except for secondary bacterial infection of the vesicles. In adults, pneumonia is the most common complication, and this may be extremely serious.

Reye's syndrome is a serious and often fatal complication of some acute viral infections, notably influenza. This syndrome is usually seen in children and closely follows the fever and other symptoms of the viral infection itself. In addition to fever, there is usually nausea and vomiting, along with a sudden change in mental status. Forgetfulness, lethargy, and disorientation may quickly progress to coma and seizures. Although the cause of this syndrome is not clearly understood, there may be some relationship between acute viral infections such as flu or chicken pox and the use of aspirin. *Avoid treating any acute viral illness in your child with aspirin.*

WHEN TO BE CONCERNED

Anytime your child has a high temperature (over 101 degrees Fahrenheit rectally) lasting longer than two days, arrange for a medical evaluation, even in the absence of other symptoms. If there are other symptoms such as cough, rash, diarrhea, headache, neck stiffness, or lethargy, your child needs *immediate* attention. When fever persists longer than a week, it's more likely due to a bacterial than a viral infection. After two weeks, consider more serious causes.

Although measles is usually not serious, complications can include pneumonia (especially in infants) as well as bacterial ear and throat infections. Chicken pox is likewise usually without complications. Bacterial infection of the vesicles may occur when care is not taken.

Mumps virus is the most common cause of aseptic meningitis (an inflammation of the lining of the brain) in childhood. Mumps symptoms include fever, headache, neck stiffness, and nausea with vomiting. Symptoms usually resolve without long-term complications. Significant abdominal pain is a symptom of mumps infection that suggests inflammation of the pancreas as a complication (*see* Abdominal Cramping and Distension). Mumps infecting the testicles (orchitis) can cause sterility.

Anytime your child has an acute viral infection such as measles, mumps, flu, or chicken pox, you must regard any signs of lethargy, forgetfulness, or other change in mental status as a medical emergency. Don't simply blame these mental changes on your child's run-down condition from the virus.

TREATMENT

The most effective treatment for measles is prevention through immunization. Several vaccines are available and provide full immunity. Your child should be vaccinated at 15 months (*see* immunization schedule in Positive Health Care, Part I). Treatment of the disease itself is largely symptomatic, with bed rest, isolation, and increased fluids. Also, protect your child from exposure to bacterial infections during a bout with measles.

Mumps can be prevented effectively through immunization. Once your doctor diagnoses mumps, the virus itself is best treated symptomatically. He'll recommend rest, fluids, and testicular support if orchitis develops, as well as other drugs for more serious complications.

Your child's doctor will ordinarily have little difficulty diagnosing chicken pox. He'll probably recommend symptomatic treatment

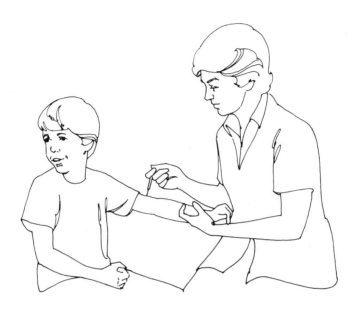

consisting of fluids, antihistamines to control your child's itching, and acetaminophen (Tylenol) to lower the temperature. A good suggestion is to keep your child's nails clipped closely and keep his hands especially clean to prevent bacterial infection of the scabs.

When Reye's syndrome complicates a viral infection such as chicken pox, immediate hospitalization with intensive medical support and management is urgent.

CALL YOUR DOCTOR WHEN:

- your child has a high temperature (over 101 degrees Fahrenheit rectally) lasting longer than two days.
- your child has any symptoms of cough, rash, headache, neck stiffness, or lethargy (call immediately).
- your child complains of swelling of the salivary glands under the jaws.
- you suspect any bacterial complication of a routine viral infection.

RASHES IN INFANTS AND CHILDREN

DESCRIPTION

Rashes in infants and children are often the same as in adults, usually with the same characteristic appearances. Many localized skin irritations may have itching (*see* Itching) as their main symptom. These include fungal infections, poison ivy, insect bites, lice, and scabies. Also, viral infections such as measles and chicken pox often cause generalized rashes (*see* Generalized Rashes). Still other rashes, such as syphilis, thrush, and herpes, more commonly affect the mucous membranes (*see* Irritation of the Mucous Membranes). Like an adult, your infant or child may also develop an abscess or other localized pockets of infection such as acne, a boil, or a furuncle (*see* Other Skin Irritations).

As if these conditions were not enough, still other rashes are even more common in infants and children. Diaper rash is a skin inflammation (dermatitis) caused by prolonged contact between your child's skin and his urine and feces. The urea and intestinal enzymes cause a reddening and thickening of the skin. After three or four days, this condition often becomes complicated by a yeast infection.

Seborrhea is a red, scaly inflammation of the skin, especially around the face and scalp, that usually occurs either in the newborn or at puberty. Most commonly, you'll find that your baby has developed a thick, yellowish crust on his scalp that may also involve his face. Having your child's doctor check any persistent rash is a good idea so that you don't confuse this condition with an allergic skin reaction or even with impetigo.

Impetigo is a highly contagious bacterial skin infection especially common in babies and children. It is caused by staph alone or by both staph and strep bacteria and occurs mainly on the arms, legs, and face. The rash usually starts as red patches on the face, which quickly turn to blisters. These enlarge and drain a yellowish liquid that forms crusts. Itching is common, and scratching may spread the infection.

WHEN TO BE CONCERNED

Diaper rash is a common problem in infants and generally responds well to careful hygiene and local treatment. If this condition persists for several days and the skin becomes beefy-red, suspect a yeast infection.

Generally, the pediatrician should check any persistent rash on the child's scalp or face. These rashes are commonly seborrhea during the first few months of life, but they may also be due to allergy or impetigo. Any skin irritation may lead to a serious bacterial infection if it is not properly managed. If your child develops pustules or crusty yellow sores on his face, arms, and legs, call the doctor. If impetigo is not treated promptly, it can become a widespread and life-threatening infection.

TREATMENT

Changing your infant's diapers frequently will prevent prolonged contact of urine and stool with his skin. Avoid using rubber or plastic pants since these prevent evaporation of moisture and worsen the irritation by promoting penetration into the skin. When you use talcum powder regularly, it will help absorb moisture. Avoid using cornstarch since this encourages yeast infections. If your child's doctor suspects a yeast infection, he may prescribe Nystatin cream and possibly also cortisone cream in severe cases.

If your child has seborrhea, treatment will depend on the location and severity of the condition. The pediatrician may recommend various shampoos to control the scaling skin (dandruff) and possibly cortisone creams in severe cases.

Because impetigo is contagious, never share towels or facecloths with someone who is infected. The crusts should be soaked in warm water and washed off with antiseptic soap. Consult your child's doctor to determine if antibiotics are indicated. Antibiotic creams and lotions are usually effective once the crusts have been removed. For severe cases, oral antibiotics may be prescribed.

CALL YOUR DOCTOR WHEN:

- your child has a persistent rash around his genital and rectal area that becomes beefy-red or does not respond to careful hygiene.
- your child has an oily, red, scaling rash on his scalp or face.
- your child has blisters or crusty yellow sores on his face, arms, or legs.

COUGH AND/OR SHORTNESS OF BREATH IN INFANTS AND CHILDREN

DESCRIPTION

A persistent cough or shortness of breath in an infant or child can be a serious symptom that requires *immediate* medical evaluation. Your child's cough is a reflex defense mechanism for removing irritants from his airways. It is important to determine the cause of any persistent cough (*see* Cough and/or Shortness of Breath). Also, other symptoms associated with your child's cough may be helpful in determining its cause. The cough may be wet or dry and may be associated with a fever, shortness of breath, lethargy, or a rash. Among other things, a cough (*see* Cough) is most commonly caused by an allergy or a bacterial or a viral infection.

Croup is an acute viral inflammation of the upper and lower respiratory tracts. It usually occurs between the ages of six months and three years. It is more serious than most other viral infections and may quickly become life threatening.

Your young child will usually develop croup gradually following a typical upper respiratory viral infection. He may have a slight fever, along with a spasmodic cough, hoarseness, and wheezing. As your child's windpipe becomes swollen and obstructed, you may notice a harsh sound (stridor) as he has increasing difficulty in exhaling. Your child may quickly become very short of breath and anxious as he is unable to get enough oxygen.

Unlike adults, who commonly develop pneumonia localized in one lobe of their lung, infants and children tend to develop a more widespread infection that is more likely to block their airways. As with many other illnesses in infants and small children, pneumonia usually develops suddenly, often following an upper respiratory infection. There will often be an associated fever, cough, and rapid heartbeat, especially in infants. An older child may also complain of some shortness of breath and chest pain.

WHEN TO BE CONCERNED

Anytime your child develops any hoarseness or shortness of breath associated with a viral illness, he requires *immediate* medical attention. The main complication of croup is asphyxia from swelling and blockage of your child's airway. Croup, with or without a fever, may quickly become a life-threatening condition. Even if you suspect this is the cause of your child's symptoms, don't overlook other possibilities. Has your child swallowed some small object that has stuck in his windpipe? Is there an abscess or other infection blocking his throat or larynx? As symptoms of breathlessness become more severe, don't delay medical care while you wait for an improvement.

If your infant or child develops a fever with a cough and shortness of breath after an upper respiratory infection, suspect pneumonia. Pneumonia in infants is commonly caused by both viruses and bacteria and is always serious. If your child is short of breath or is coughing up yellowish-green sputum or bright red blood, *immediate* medical care is urgent. Neck stiffness associated with an upper respiratory infection or pneumonia may indicate an early case of meningitis and also requires *immediate* medical care. Older children with pneumonia may complain of chest pain and shortness of breath as well. Other complications of pneumonia may include lung abscesses, shock, and heart failure.

TREATMENT

If you are at home or far from emergency medical care, mist or steam inhalation from a vaporizer or from a hot shower may help to relieve your child's symptoms of croup. Try to keep him relaxed. Restlessness is a sign that he is not getting enough oxygen. Provide lots of fluids for him to drink.

If your child doesn't respond promptly to these simple measures, get him to an emergency medical facility *immediately*. Various medications are available that may help to reduce his airway obstruction. An emergency tracheotomy, to provide an airway, may be required in serious cases where the windpipe closes quickly and cuts off the supply of oxygen. This emergency procedure can be done best in a properly equipped facility by specially trained personnel.

Pneumonia caused by both viruses and bacteria usually requires hospitalization and intensive medical management. If you suspect this diagnosis, don't waste valuable time attempting home treatment. The doctor will take a thorough medical history and carefully examine your child. He'll need to be certain that there is no other underlying cause for his symptoms and no other complications. He will likely request blood tests as well as a chest X-ray to confirm his diagnosis. Your child's sputum may be cultured to determine the exact cause of his pneumonia. Besides recommending rest and lots of fluids, the doctor will probably prescribe antibiotics for most cases of pneumonia.

CALL YOUR DOCTOR WHEN:

- your child develops any shortness of breath, with or without a fever.
- your child develops a cough and a high fever following a mild respiratory infection.

EARACHES IN CHILDREN

DESCRIPTION

In infants and children, middle ear infections are the most common cause of earache (*see* Earache). Young children are more commonly affected because they get more colds and their ear canals are shorter. Traumatic injuries to the canal or eardrum and foreign objects lodged in the canal also commonly cause earache. Although your infant or young child will be unable to describe an earache, you'll notice his increased irritability, difficulty in sleeping, or constant tugging at his ear.

Usually an earache caused by infection (*see* Ear Infections) will be associated with fever, a discharge from the canal (*see* Bleeding or Discharge from the Ear), or symptoms of a cold. If your child's earache is caused by an injury or a foreign object lodged in the canal, there may be no symptoms or only scanty bleeding.

WHEN TO BE CONCERNED

If your young child complains of ear pain or is especially irritable and tugs repeatedly on his ear, suspect an earache. If symptoms of a cold and fever are present, a middle ear infection is a good possibility. A thick, yellowish drainage from the canal makes an outer ear infection more likely. Blood from the canal is a serious sign that may indicate a perforated eardrum or other serious injury. If your child has been near small toys or sharp objects like a pencil, suspect a foreign body or other traumatic injury.

TREATMENT

Whatever the cause, your child's earache deserves prompt medical evaluation. Don't begin home treatment without a doctor's recommendation. Avoid inserting cotton swabs or other foreign objects into the ear and don't wash or rinse the ear on your own. You may only spread an infection or push a foreign object farther into the canal.

The pediatrician will carefully examine the canal for foreign bodies or signs of infection. There are special instruments and techniques he can use to remove small objects. He'll also check the eardrum for a perforation or an infection behind it. If the canal is infected, a culture may be taken and antibiotics prescribed. A punctured eardrum requires careful evaluation and follow-up to assure proper healing without complications.

CALL YOUR DOCTOR WHEN:

• you suspect that your infant or small child has ear pain from any cause.

PART V

COMMON MEDICAL EMERGENCIES

Chapter 16

Emergency Situations

CARDIAC ARREST

DESCRIPTION

Cardiac arrest resulting from a heart attack or from an accident is probably the most frequent life-threatening emergency today. Most often cardiac arrest is the result of a major acute blockage that aggravates a chronic obstruction of the coronary arteries supplying blood to the heart. Sometimes this obstruction becomes so severe that the heart is unable to get enough oxygen-carrying blood. In many cases, a particular type of chest pain (angina) (*see* Chest Pain) is a warning sign of this chronic obstruction. Other times there is no warning before a heart attack (myocardial infarction), and a portion of the heart muscle dies as a result. Although most heart attacks do not result in cardiac arrest, they almost always cause permanent damage to the heart muscle.

A cardiac arrest from any cause is basically a *total* loss of heart function due either to the complete cessation of the heartbeat or to the loss of any effective heart rhythm. Besides heart attacks, some other causes of cardiac arrest include choking (*see* Choking), drowning (*see* Drowning), and electric shock (*see* Electric Shock). Cardiac arrest is a medical emergency since permanent brain damage can result in as few as four or five minutes. Cardiopulmonary resuscitation (CPR) performed by someone skilled in this technique can maintain life until emergency medical treatment arrives.

Besides those who suffer cardiac arrest from other accidents, over 1.5 million people a year have heart attacks, and almost half of these die. About half of these deaths occur before victims ever reach a hospital. It is estimated that at least 100,000 of these lives could be saved each year through the prompt use of CPR.

WHEN TO BE CONCERNED

Anytime you witness someone suddenly lose consciousness, you must suspect a cardiac arrest. Although this medical emergency may occur in either sex at any age, older men and individuals with a history of angina or other heart disease are at the greatest risk. If an individual suddenly loses consciousness while eating, you should also suspect choking (*see* Choking) as the underlying cause.

When sudden loss of consciousness follows a poisoning, a drowning, or an electrical shock, you should also suspect a cardiac arrest as the cause. Learn and practice the techniques of cardiopulmonary resuscitation before an emergency arises. Prompt action can be lifesaving since brain damage occurs in a matter of minutes.

Promptly check for signs of cardiac and/or respiratory failure. These signs include loss of consciousness, absent pulse, absent breathing, dilated pupils, and cool, pale skin with a bluish cast (cyanosis). If any of these signs are present, summon help if nearby and begin CPR *immediately*.

TREATMENT

The only effective treatment for a cardiac arrest is to begin CPR *immediately*. Everyone from teenagers to senior citizens should be sure to take the time to learn CPR. Regardless of its cause, cardiac arrest requires immediate attention to restoring the circulatory and respiratory function of the heart and lungs.

If you witness a cardiac arrest or come upon an unconscious patient, don't waste time trying to determine the underlying cause of the problem. Every second is vital! If the cardiac arrest is the result of an electric shock, carefully remove the victim (without directly touching him) from the source of the current. If you suspect poisoning as the cause of the cardiac arrest, don't attempt to induce vomiting or otherwise treat the poisoning. Begin CPR immediately!

Use the techniques of CPR you've learned to determine if respiration and circulatory function has ceased. A victim in cardiac arrest will rapidly stop breathing. Similarly, a drowning victim who is unable to breathe will quickly suffer cardiac arrest. Begin to aerate the lungs as soon as possible, and begin CPR as soon as a solid surface is available to support the victim's chest.

Careful training is essential to master these CPR techniques, and today this training is widely available at your local YMCA, YWCA, Red Cross, and local health clubs.

SUSPECT A CARDIAC ARREST AND BEGIN CPR WHEN:

- you witness a victim suddenly lose consciousness and you are unable to detect a pulse and/or respiration (*have someone call for help immediately*).
- a victim loses consciousness following an electrical shock, a near drowning, or a poisoning.
- you find an unconscious victim without detectable pulse or respiration (*have someone call for help immediately*).

CHOKING

DESCRIPTION

Most people don't realize that choking can be a life-threatening emergency. Statistics show that this is one of the leading causes of accidental death in the United States and that it actually causes more deaths than either firearms or airline accidents. Both young children and adults are often victims. Choking causes brain damage and death in a matter of minutes because it prevents breathing, cutting off oxygen to the lungs. This lack of oxygen often leads to loss of consciousness and cardiac arrest (*see* Cardiac Arrest).

Choking occurs so easily because your windpipe (trachea) opens right behind the tongue near the beginning of your esophagus. When you swallow food or drink, a reflex normally closes off your trachea, preventing any blockage of your airway. Sometimes the trachea fails to close properly and the food goes "down the wrong tube." Usually, this merely causes a spasmodic cough reflex, forcing the particle out. But sometimes a large piece of food becomes wedged in the trachea, totally obstructing the victim's airway. This prevents oxygen from reaching the lungs and causes asphyxiation. Because permanent brain damage and cardiac arrest occur in a matter of minutes, it is essential that you learn emergency techniques (*see* Heimlich Maneuver) to aid such a victim.

WHEN TO BE CONCERNED

If you witness a victim suddenly lose consciousness while eating, suspect choking as a possible cause. Choking is usually caused when the victim's main airway (trachea) becomes blocked with a foreign object, often a large piece of food. Although other things, such as cardiac arrest or a stroke, may cause a sudden loss of consciousness, a choking victim may be unable to talk, cough, or even breathe immediately after the accident.

A diner who suddenly loses consciousness while talking or laughing has very likely suffered an acute airway obstruction. Choking is even more likely to occur in diners who have consumed significant amounts of alcohol. This dulls their senses and suppresses their normal protective cough reflex. Often a choking victim will appear

HEIMLICH MANEUVER

With the Victim Sitting or Standing:

1. Place your fist with the thumb against the victim's abdomen, above the navel and below the ribcage.

2. Grasp the fist with your other hand and press it upward into the abdomen with a sharp thrust.

3. Stand behind the victim if he is standing and kneel if he is sitting.

4. You may need to repeat this maneuver several times.

With the Victim Lying on His Back:

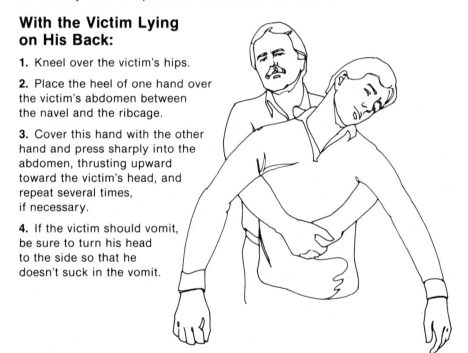

1. Kneel over the victim's hips.

2. Place the heel of one hand over the victim's abdomen between the navel and the ribcage.

3. Cover this hand with the other hand and press sharply into the abdomen, thrusting upward toward the victim's head, and repeat several times, if necessary.

4. If the victim should vomit, be sure to turn his head to the side so that he doesn't suck in the vomit.

If the victim is an infant or small child, use your forefinger and middle finger instead of a fist to apply the thrust. If you are unable to reach around an obese victim, first place him on his back. If you are a victim of choking, you may try this technique on yourself if you are alone or nobody is capable of performing the maneuver.

panicky, turn bluish, and grasp at his throat before losing consciousness. If the victim is still able to cough, complete airway obstruction is unlikely. Allow a moment for him to cough up the obstructing object on his own before you attempt a rescue.

TREATMENT

The best treatment for choking as well as for most other accidents is prevention. Following a few simple rules would prevent most deaths caused by choking. Never talk or laugh with food in your mouth. Avoid excessive alcohol, especially before eating. Take small bites and chew your food carefully. Be especially careful if you wear dentures. Also, never eat when you're out of breath or when you are exercising vigorously. Finally, be especially careful with infants and small children. Expect them to put everything nearby in their mouths, including toys, buttons, coins, etc.

Once you recognize that a person is choking, especially if he or she has lost consciousness, you have only a minute or two in which to act. Your prompt response and knowledge of a technique called the Heimlich Maneuver may well save a life. This technique can usually be taught by your local YMCA, YWCA, or Red Cross, or by your doctor. Even children have successfully used this technique to save siblings who were choking. Also, everyone should know and recognize the "universal choking sign." This is the sign that a choking victim should use to attract the attention of a nearby rescuer. It consists of grasping the throat with the right hand.

SUSPECT CHOKING AND PERFORM THE HEIMLICH MANEUVER WHEN:

- you see a victim who is eating suddenly become unable to cough or talk and begin to turn bluish (*have someone call for help immediately*).
- you see a victim give you the "universal choking sign" (*have someone call for help immediately*).
- you find an unconscious victim with a detectable pulse and no respiration and you suspect choking (in performing CPR following a cardiac arrest, the first step must always be to establish a clear airway) (*have someone call for help immediately*).

LACERATIONS

DESCRIPTION

Laceration is a general term for any injury in which there is a ragged tearing of your tissues. These always result from a traumatic injury and are often accompanied by bruises (contusions), abrasions, and incised wounds (cuts).

WHEN TO BE CONCERNED

If your laceration is large, or if you have significant bruising, damage to surrounding tissues, or persistent bleeding, seek *immediate* care. Lacerations often contain dead tissue and foreign matter that must be removed to prevent infection and to ensure proper healing.

Extensive lacerations are often associated with damage to surrounding structures. This damage may include severed veins and arteries, nerve damage, and injuries to tendons and ligaments. If your wound is "dirty," you are at high risk for infection. If the circulation to your injured tissue is inadequate, you may develop gangrene. Broken or dislocated bones, as well as torn tendons and ligaments, must be treated properly to prevent long-term disability.

TREATMENT

If you are far from an emergency facility, direct your immediate attention at controlling significant bleeding and preventing infection. To stop external bleeding effectively, apply pressure directly to the wound. Calm the victim, have him lie down, and elevate the injured extremity. Quickly try to remove large fragments from the wound. It is urgent that you stop the bleeding immediately, using a clean pad, a rag, or even your fingers. Compress the wound firmly. If the bleeding persists, use a tourniquet intermittently to put pressure over the artery supplying the wounded area. Learn these main "pressure points" from a first-aid manual or course before an emergency arises.

If you have an extensive laceration, don't attempt any other treatment. Cover the injured area with a clean dressing and go to the hospital as soon as possible. Most significant lacerations require prompt medical attention. Injuries that are dirty and have foreign bodies embedded in them must be cleaned with sterile surgical instruments. Dead tissue and substances such as cinders and glass must be removed carefully since they promote infection. Often, bleeding from damage to major blood vessels is persistent and requires surgical attention. Bone, ligament, and tendon damage near the injury must be repaired. Your doctor will need to evaluate your immunization status to determine if your immunity to tetanus is adequate.

CALL YOUR DOCTOR WHEN:

- you have any significant bleeding as a result of a laceration (call immediately).
- your wound is "dirty" and contains foreign matter or injured tissue.
- you have any numbness or tingling in an extremity after a laceration.
- you have severe pain or are unable to move an extremity after an injury.

BURNS

DESCRIPTION

A burn is an injury caused by thermal, electrical, or chemical agents. Your skin ordinarily protects your body from infection and regulates body temperature. A burn destroys this protection. The terms first, second, and third degree indicate the degree of tissue damage from a burn.

First degree—only the outer layer (epidermis) is affected, and the skin becomes red and tender. Most sun overexposure causes first degree burns.

Second degree—both the epidermis and underlying layer (dermis) are burned, and redness and blistering occur with significant pain. Severe sunburn may cause second-degree burns.

Third degree—the most serious burns damage the full depth of skin as well as underlying tissues, including nerve endings. These burns are usually the least painful but may require skin grafting.

WHEN TO BE CONCERNED

The degree (first, second, or third) of your burn and the percentage of skin surface affected indicate the severity. But age is also important since burns are more serious in the very young and very old. Besides skin damage, other problems such as smoke inhalation are often associated with burns. Infection resulting from burns is a major complication, especially in already debilitated patients such as diabetics and the elderly.

TREATMENT

As with poisonings and many other accidents, an ounce of prevention is worth a pound of cure. Don't allow small children near hot objects in the kitchen or bath. Keep flammable liquids in a safe place. Avoid overloading electrical outlets and keep children away from wiring. Place smoke detectors throughout your house. In case of fire, get everyone out of the house first, then call the fire department.

Home treatment for minor first-degree burns (including sunburn) consists of cold packs. Healing will usually occur within a week.

More severe burns with redness and blistering should have prompt medical attention. In general, the primary objective with all burns is prevention of infection and promotion of fast wound healing. Most large cities have special hospital burn units staffed with specialists in burn care.

CALL YOUR DOCTOR WHEN:

• you have a burn that has caused any blistering of the skin.

DROWNING

DESCRIPTION

Drowning causes over 7,000 accidental deaths in this country each year. Many could be prevented with proper safety precautions, prompt rescue, and use of cardiopulmonary resuscitation (CPR) (*see* Cardiac Arrest). Nowadays, training programs in CPR are available from many organizations, including local health departments, and the Red Cross.

Drowning is not simply caused by the lungs filling with water. Many different mechanisms may cause death. Salt water and fresh water each cause different problems. When fresh water is taken into the lungs, it dilutes and destroys blood cells and disrupts the normal chemical balance, resulting in heart abnormalities and death. Salt water taken into the lungs actually draws in body water and causes death from lack of oxygen.

WHEN TO BE CONCERNED

When you see someone drowning, quickly assess the situation. Is the victim unconscious or struggling to keep afloat? Is he trapped in some way? Are you skilled in lifesaving? What other help is available? Unskilled rescuers themselves often drown. Conscious victims can sometimes be saved by using a float or rope.

Once a victim has been rescued, quickly evaluate his condition. Use your CPR training to be sure he has an adequate airway and circulation or promptly begin resuscitation efforts. If no heartbeat or pulse is present, begin cardiac massage. If the victim isn't breathing, don't waste time trying to remove water from the lungs or stomach. Begin resuscitation *immediately!* If the victim has an adequate heartbeat and spontaneous respirations at the time of rescue, recovery is likely.

TREATMENT

Your most urgent task with any drowning victim is restoring oxygen and reestablishing blood circulation. If possible, begin CPR even before removing the victim from the water. Get air into the victim's lungs *immediately.*

Allow trained help to take over when it arrives. All victims require hospitalization and support to prevent later complications, which include heart and lung problems, chemical imbalances, and infections.

CALL YOUR DOCTOR WHEN:

- anyone has suffered a near drowning or has taken significant amounts of water into the lungs or stomach.

ELECTRICAL SHOCK

DESCRIPTION

While electrical shock is not as common a cause of injury and death as other accidents, many people underestimate the danger from small household appliances. Electrical shock usually causes injury in three ways. Most seriously, a shock can affect the breathing center in the brain and the heart rhythm, causing failure of respiration and circulation. Also, an electrical current can cause severe burns (*see* Burns).

To a large extent, the injury from an electrical shock depends on the circumstances. Besides the strength of the current, the contact between the victim and the ground is important. Most important is avoiding any contact with electrical appliances when your hands are wet or when you are standing in water. Children are especially vulnerable to electrical accidents from electrical outlets or from chewing on wires.

WHEN TO BE CONCERNED

When a person has sustained an electrical shock, there may be a loss of consciousness. This situation is urgent since it is likely due to a cessation of respiration and heartbeat. In this situation, immediate cardiopulmonary resuscitation (CPR) (*see* Cardiac Arrest) may be lifesaving. If there is an electrical burn, *immediate* evaluation is required to assess the extent of tissue damage and prevent secondary infection. Any victim of a severe electrical shock (with or without loss of consciousness) or a burn requires *immediate* care.

TREATMENT

The best treatment for electrical shock is prevention. Avoid any combination of electricity with water and keep all appliances and wiring in good repair. Learn CPR techniques! When a victim of electrical shock has lost consciousness, suspect cardiac and respiratory arrest. Carefully remove the victim from the electrical source, avoiding contact yourself. Begin CPR *immediately* and summon help. *Emergency medical care is urgently needed.*

After an electrical burn, damage to underlying tissues and organs must be evaluated carefully. Dead tissue should be removed. As with other burns, treatment should be aimed at preventing infection and promoting healing.

CALL YOUR DOCTOR WHEN:

- someone has sustained a severe electrical shock with or without a loss of consciousness or a burn.

BLEEDING EMERGENCIES

DESCRIPTION

Ordinarily, external bleeding (*see* Bleeding or Abnormal Bruising *and* Lacerations) from a minor cut, hemorrhoids, or an abrasion is not serious. Usually, such bleeding comes from small veins beneath the surface of your skin. When these blood vessels are torn, they normally contract, and elements in your blood form a clot that plugs the wound. In severe injuries, when large veins or arteries are cut or when certain clotting factors in your blood are missing, a clot may be unable to form and rapid blood loss may occur. An adult may go into shock from the loss of as little as 1½ pints of blood and a child from as little as ½ pint. This loss can be fatal if emergency action is not taken to stop it.

Less obvious *internal* bleeding may result from such things as a serious abdominal injury, a chest injury, an ulcer, or a tumor in the gastrointestinal tract (*see* Nausea and Vomiting). This type of bleeding can be just as serious as external bleeding and likewise requires emergency medical care.

WHEN TO BE CONCERNED

A major external blood loss is usually obvious, but sometimes very heavy menstrual bleeding or chronically bleeding hemorrhoids can fool you. Seek *immediate* medical attention whenever you suspect any blood loss that amounts to more than two or three tablespoons over a 24-hour period. Other clues to serious blood loss are cold, clammy skin; a rapid and weak pulse; weakness; dilated pupils; and dizziness, especially when standing.

Internal bleeding is more difficult to detect, especially when it doesn't follow an injury and occurs gradually. The symptoms mentioned above should make you suspicious. After an injury, hemorrhage into the abdominal cavity may occur from a torn blood vessel or from a ruptured spleen or other organ.

Fractures, especially of the thigh bone (femur), also commonly cause significant blood loss into the surrounding tissues. Serious hemorrhage into the gastrointestinal tract may result from an ulcer, a tumor in the stomach or colon, or, in alcoholics, from liver disease (cirrhosis) and ruptured blood vessels in the esophagus. Suspect significant gastrointestinal bleeding in anyone with a history of ulcer disease or alcohol abuse, when any of the above symptoms are present, or when there is bright red blood or tarry black stool from the rectum (*see* Rectal Pain and Bleeding).

TREATMENT

To stop external bleeding effectively, apply pressure directly to the wound. Calm the victim, have him lie down, and elevate the injured extremity. Quickly try to remove large fragments from the wound. It is urgent that you stop the bleeding immediately, using a clean pad, a rag, or even your fingers. Compress the wound firmly. If the bleeding persists, use a tourniquet intermittently to put pressure over the artery supplying the wounded area. Learn these main "pressure points" from a first-aid manual or course before an emergency arises.

Prompt suspicion and recognition of internal bleeding is urgent. Any internal bleeding requires *immediate* medical evaluation, followed by fluid and blood replacement and emergency surgical repair of the source of the hemorrhage.

CALL YOUR DOCTOR WHEN:

- you suspect a blood loss of more than two or three tablespoons from any source in a 24-hour period.
- you have external bleeding from any cause that persists despite efforts to stop it.

- you suspect internal bleeding from any cause (*call immediately*).
- you experience symptoms of weakness, dizziness, rapid pulse, or cold and clammy skin, especially following any injury (*call immediately*).

POISONING

DESCRIPTION

Many common substances in your environment may be poisons when abused or misused. Drugs, plant and insect sprays, cosmetics, detergents, and hundreds of other household articles can cause illness or possibly death. The care you give during the first few minutes following a poisoning may make the difference between life and death. Because of the many different toxic substances in our environment and the different treatments they require, a national network of Poison Control Centers has been set up. These centers maintain detailed records of the ingredients in all dangerous products and are especially equipped to handle all types of poisoning cases. Learn the location and phone number of your nearest Poison Control Center and keep it handy for an emergency.

Although most poisons are taken in by mouth, poisons may also enter your body by inhalation or by absorption or injection (from insect or snake bites) through your skin. Once a poison enters your system, it may cause harm in several different ways. Poisons such as acids or lye can actually cause severe burns and scarring of tissues. Many types of sleeping pills and alcohol depress your brain and can slow or stop respiration and other brain functions. Other drugs have an opposite stimulant effect, causing rapid blood pressure increases as well as strokes and acute psychoses. Other poisons, such as carbon monoxide and cyanide, prevent the blood from carrying oxygen to the tissues, causing asphyxiation. Still others may cause paralysis.

WHEN TO BE CONCERNED

Various poisons act in many different ways, producing a variety of symptoms. Suspect acute poisoning when contact with any substance results in mental changes such as drowsiness, seizures, or coma.

Likewise, sudden onset of breathing difficulty or shortness of breath can be a symptom of poisoning. Ingestion of acid or lye may cause severe burning in the esophagus and stomach, along with vomiting.

Often clues from the victim's surroundings will indicate the cause of poisoning. Empty bottles from drugs or chemicals may be present. Gas or odors from various poisons may be detectable. If the poison is a corrosive such as acid or lye, there may be stains or burns around the victim's mouth and lips. Sometimes the source of poisoning may not be so obvious, as when an infant absorbs poisonous cleaning materials from his clothes or linens. Always try to determine the cause of the poisoning if possible, but never delay treatment while trying to find a specific antidote.

TREATMENT

The best treatment for poisoning is to prevent it. Avoid keeping dangerous substances where they can be reached by children. Clearly label all chemicals and never store them in food containers. Never take a medicine in the dark and never take someone else's medication. Keep gas and kerosene heaters and appliances in proper working condition. Never run a gasoline generator or an automobile engine in a poorly ventilated area.

When you suspect that a poisoning has occurred, quickly analyze the situation. If the poison appears to be a corrosive such as acid or lye or a petroleum product like cleaning fluid, try to neutralize it as soon as possible. For acids, substances such as limewater, diluted milk of magnesia, or a baking soda solution are recommended. Alkali poisons (lye-based drain openers, for example) should be neutralized with large amounts of orange or lemon juice or dilute vinegar. Experts generally discourage a victim from vomiting these poisons since this may cause further irritation to the lungs.

Generally, if the poison is noncorrosive, such as sleeping pills, prompt evacuation of the stomach contents is the best early treatment. Several glasses of soapy water, baking soda solution, or preferably syrup of ipecac will usually induce vomiting. Fill the stomach with water after giving these substances. In all poisoning cases, be sure the victim does not suck the vomited substances into his lungs. Don't delay while you wait for your home treatment to work. Call the Poison Control Center and rush the victim to the nearest emergency room. Try to bring a sample of the poison or some of the stomach contents along with the victim so that the type of poison can be determined.

CALL YOUR POISON CONTROL CENTER AND SEEK EMERGENCY CARE WHEN:

- you suspect that someone has been poisoned and you need specific instructions (*call immediately*).
- you suspect that someone is a victim of a snake bite or may be having an allergic reaction to an insect bite (*call immediately*).

FROSTBITE

DESCRIPTION

Prolonged exposure to dry cold (temperatures well below freezing) causes frostbite and, in severe cases, loss of consciousness and death. Frostbite most commonly occurs on your ears, nose, hands, and feet, especially if your circulation is already poor. Your involved fingers or toes first appear white and frozen. Once you reach medical care the frostbitten area may appear red and swollen as thawing begins. The tissue may be blistered, but gangrene at this early stage is rare.

Milder frostbite may not permanently damage your tissues. More severe cases may cause damage similar to that in burns. This mostly occurs from clots blocking your capillary circulation. If you've had frostbite in the past, you may be especially sensitive to cold and new tissue damage.

WHEN TO BE CONCERNED

Frostbite is one medical emergency for which the cause is known. Be concerned if the involved part has become numb, hard, cold, and pale. Once your circulation has been disrupted for a prolonged period of time, gangrene may begin to develop. In addition to localized symptoms of frostbite, severe overexposure to cold may result in significant mental changes such as confusion, hallucinations, loss of consciousness, and a slowed heartbeat.

TREATMENT

Experts now believe that rapid is far more effective than slow rewarming. Remove any wet or restrictive clothing. Avoid massaging a frostbitten extremity or breaking blisters that form. A warm bath (at 100 degrees Fahrenheit), hot drinks, and heating pads are recommended. Dry your skin after baths to prevent injury and be careful to avoid infecting any damaged tissue.

If you suspect frostbite, seek *immediate* medical attention. After rewarming, your doctor will remove the dead tissue and assess the damage. He'll check your pulse and the capillary circulation to the injured areas. If complications of infection are suspected, antibiotics may be prescribed and the area dressed as a burn injury. Severe cases require hospitalization and intravenous medications to improve capillary circulation.

CALL YOUR DOCTOR WHEN:

• you have any persistent numbness of your extremities following exposure to cold.

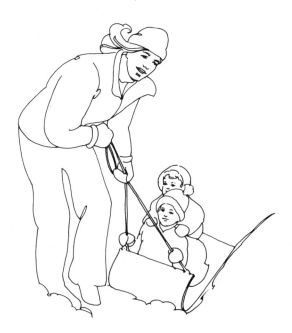

PSYCHIATRIC EMERGENCIES

DESCRIPTION

It's normal to feel down (*see* Personality Change) or anxious (*see* Anxiety) from time to time. Life in today's fast-paced, complex society is full of stresses that may make coping seem difficult. Fortunately, these feelings of depression and anxiety are usually brief and self-limited. However, if they should become so intense that life seems hopeless and suicide the only way out of your problems, you must seek *immediate* medical attention. *This is a life-threatening emergency.* Likewise, if a family member's behavior suddenly changes, especially if you feel that he may be a danger to himself or others, consult your physician *immediately*.

Besides severe anxiety and depression, extreme agitation, hostility, and frank abusive or homicidal behavior seem to be increasingly evident today. Violence is now becoming a common form of conflict resolution. These abnormal behaviors are often aggravated by drug and/or alcohol dependence. To complicate matters further, medical emergencies such as acute drug reactions or infections may on occasion appear first as serious behavioral problems.

WHEN TO BE CONCERNED

Ordinarily, occasional bouts of anxiety or depression are normal human emotions, especially when they can be related to a particular situation or event. Learn to recognize the signs and symptoms of depression (*see* Common Signs and Symptoms of Depression) in yourself and those around you. When these emotions become extreme, they may even be life-threatening. Any sudden, unexplained changes in mood require *immediate* psychiatric evaluation. Always take discussions or threats about suicide seriously. Never leave any individual alone if you suspect that he or she contemplates suicide.

Sometimes extreme anxiety can be a symptom of a serious psychological disturbance. Occasionally agitated, hostile, and even homicidal people are mistaken as simply anxious. These patients are often capable of harming themselves and others and require urgent medical evaluation and treatment. Often these extreme behavior patterns are brought on or aggravated by drug reactions.

TREATMENT

Do not attempt to provide home mental health treatment to anyone whom you suspect is extremely anxious or depressed. Any significant change in mood in yourself or a loved one requires *immediate* medical evaluation. Also, sudden personality changes where agitated, hostile, or abusive behavior are displayed should not be dismissed as simply temper tantrums. These behaviors may be symptomatic of a serious underlying emotional and/or physical disorder.

CALL YOUR DOCTOR WHEN:

- you or someone close to you develops symptoms of extreme anxiety or depression.
- you or someone close to you contemplates or expresses thoughts of suicide.
- you or someone close to you displays sudden bouts of agitated, hostile, or abusive behavior.

About the Authors

Joel N. Shlian, M.D., and Deborah M. Shlian, M.D., both board-certified physicians, have been collaborating, as doctors, authors, and most recently as law students, since their marriage fifteen years ago. Joel is on the teaching faculty in the Division of Family Medicine at UCLA. Deborah is Director of Primary Care at UCLA's Student Health Service. The Shlians have coauthored several medical research articles, as well as two novels and a screenplay. They live in Los Angeles.

Index